EASY KETO IN
30 MINUTES

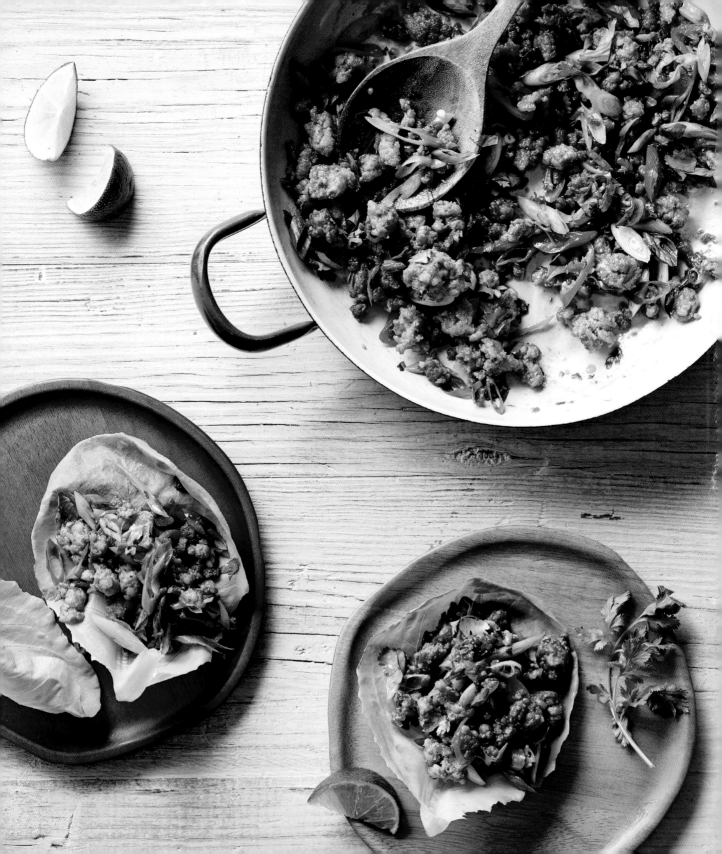

EASY KETO IN
30 MINUTES

URVASHI PITRE

PHOTOGRAPHY BY GHAZALLE BADIOZAMANI

HOUGHTON MIFFLIN HARCOURT

BOSTON   NEW YORK   2020

Copyright © 2020 by Blue Glass Jar, Inc.

Photography © 2020 by Ghazalle Badiozamani

Food styling by Monica Pierini

Prop styling by Jenna Tedesco

For information about permission to reproduce
selections from this book, write to trade.permissions@
hmhco.com or to Permissions, Houghton Mifflin
Harcourt Publishing Company, 3 Park Avenue, 19th Floor,
New York, New York 10016.

hmhbooks.com

Library of Congress Cataloging-in-Publication Data is
available.

ISBN 978-0-358-24216-1 (pbk)

ISBN 978-0-358-23777-8 (ebk)

Book design by Jennifer K. Beal Davis

Printed in China

SCP 10 9 8 7 6 5 4 3 2 1

TO MY FAMILY, WHO
STAND BEHIND ME DAILY,
AND ONLY TELL ME ONCE
A WEEK HOW BOSSY I AM.

CONTENTS

VEGETABLES

EGGS & CHEESE

CHICKEN

SEAFOOD

BEEF, PORK & LAMB

DESSERTS & DRINKS

SAUCES, DRESSINGS & SPICE MIXES

ACKNOWLEDGMENTS

It takes a village—actually, maybe sometimes two villages, even. There are so many people to thank for this book.

My family, who continue to eat all my successes and failures and give me honest feedback no matter what.

John and Diane Kasinger, who test recipes, taste recipes, and critique them for me.

Sammy and Paul Brakebill, who help me keep twosleevers.com going when I'm in the throes of recipe creation. To Sammy, I also owe thanks for (a) not being driven crazy by me, and (b) always believing in me.

Lisa Kingsley and Will Bortz, for rewriting recipes for clarity.

My agent, Stacey Glick, who is always available when I need her and who supports me in so many ways.

My editor, Justin Schwartz—our first noncrash (ish) book together! Your involvement and input really help these books come together.

Ghazalle Badiozamani and her team of accomplished stylists and helpers make my food look pretty—not just tasty. Thank you to Monica Pieroni, Krystal Rack, Jenna Tedesco, and Bridget Kenny for your great work. I so love working with you.

Thanks also to Brianna Yamashita and Samantha Simon, who help me brainstorm crazy marketing ideas, as well as the whole army at Houghton Mifflin Harcourt that helped without my even realizing it to make this book a reality.

And of course, to my fans, followers, and readers who continue to support, suggest, encourage, and make me laugh daily.

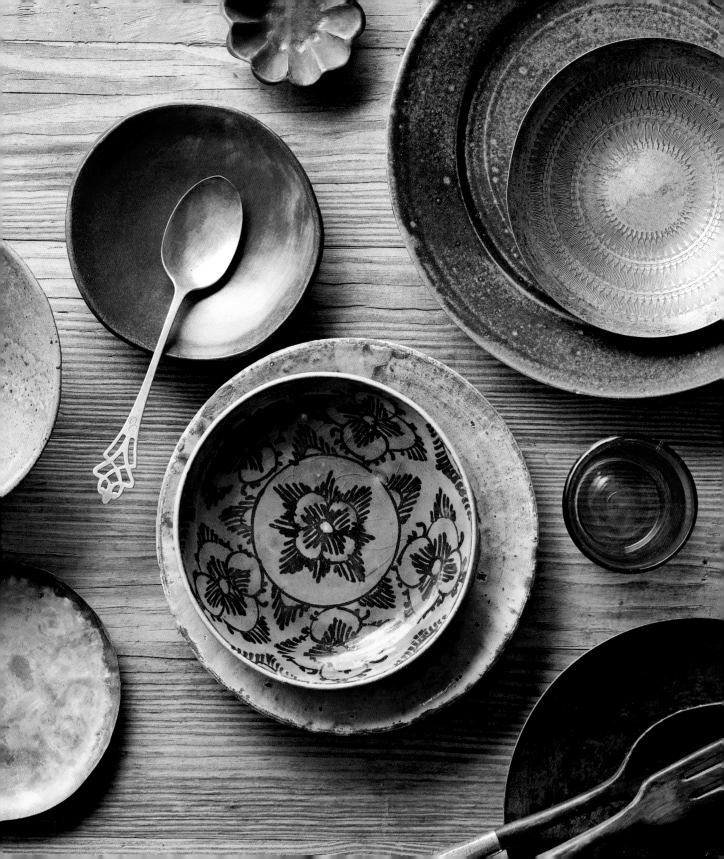

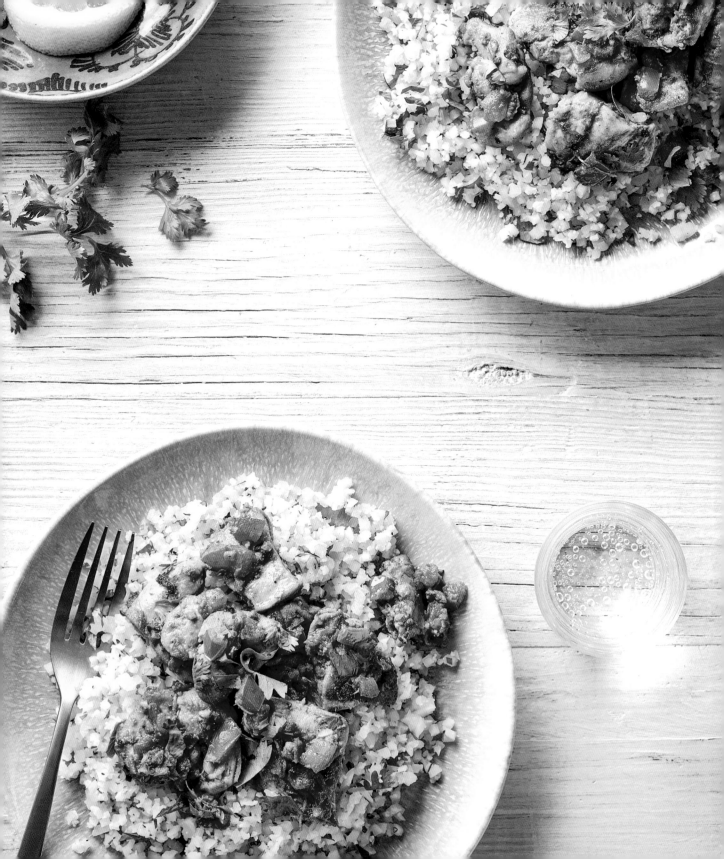

INTRODUCTION

You can be an accomplished career woman, a great mother, and the best friend ever. You can speak six languages and dance backward in high heels. But if you're overweight, chances are that's the first thing people notice about you. For many people, that's the last thing they'll notice about you as well. It's so easy to be dismissed as "less than" when you're carrying extra weight. I think this is due to the prevalent belief in our society that people are overweight because they lack self-control or discipline.

I assure you, I do not lack self-control. I am extremely disciplined. I rose to the top of my career as chief marketing information officer for a large advertising agency by dint of great discipline and a work ethic that had me working 16- to 18-hour days, in addition to trying to be a good mother. But I am quite sure that when I first walked into a room, what people probably noticed about me was the eighty extra pounds I was carrying.

The idea that those who weigh more got that way because they eat more is also well-entrenched in our belief system, so much so that people will discount the evidence before them and continue to believe the myth that "overweight = overeater," and that's why they got to be overweight. My colleagues loved going out with me for meals. Many would ask what I planned to have and order something different. They did this because they knew they would finish their food, and then they'd eat half of mine since I never finished my portion. These same people spent days on end with me on business trips, where we all spent hours together and ate together. They saw what I ate. It was less than what most of them ate.

Yet I was overweight, and they were not.

What do you want to bet that some of them thought I secretly ate late at night, in my hotel room? (For the record, I did not.) Be honest, wouldn't you have believed that?

I was never someone who ate an entire large pizza by myself. I have never polished off a cake without sharing. I have never even eaten a whole pint of ice cream by myself. I was not a binge eater. I did not eat in secret. I didn't exceed normal portions. In a society where we firmly believe in the "all calories are equal" and "expend more calories as you ingest" theories of weight loss, people will discount your behavior, and continue to believe that if you're overweight, you're eating more than those who are not overweight.

There are many other explanations for why people become overweight. In my case, the explanations were simple—but it took me years to identify them. During those years, I followed every eating style dictated by "experts." I tried vegetarian, paleo, starvation, vegan diets. I tried eating five small meals. I ate less than 800 calories a day, and during a few horrible months, I tried eating 2,500 calories a day because I was told I needed to "fuel my metabolism." I tried it all.

But the weight did not come off.

There was one thing I never tried—and that was a ketogenic diet. Part of this was my natural inclination to eat a vegetarian diet over a carnivorous diet. There is nothing wrong with a delicious vegetarian diet—unless, like me, you are extremely sensitive to carbohydrates and insulin resistant. Then, eating brown rice and beans is probably not the best for you. It certainly wasn't the best thing for me.

The other part of it was that I didn't believe it would work for me, since I had failed with so many other things. My inability to lose weight—my failure to, as I saw it—weighed on me. I hate failing; I mean, we all do, but I HATE failing! I take it very personally and I get obsessed with it, and it's . . . well, let's just say it's not pretty.

In desperation, I decided to have weight loss surgery. I felt I had exhausted every other avenue. But before I did that, I had to understand that the surgery by itself would accomplish little. By dint of enforcing fasting, it might help me in the early days after surgery. But over time, it's entirely possible to put back on the weight if you don't change your eating habits. I heard many stories from people who had put back on all—if not more of—the weight, even after surgery. Every physician I spoke to was quite clear that surgery by itself would not do the trick—I had to embrace a ketogenic diet.

My weight issues were probably linked to my untreated hypothyroidism, my extreme carb-sensitivity, and my insulin resistance. There is one way of eating that is beneficial for all these conditions—and that is a ketogenic diet.

Five years ago, once I accepted that I would have to change my diet forever, my husband and I had vertical sleeve surgery. We embraced a keto/low-carb diet, changed the way we ate all together, and accepted that this was our eating style going forward.

I still struggle with my weight every day. I still have to monitor what I eat, I still have to track, and, when I fall off the wagon, I still gain weight. I can eat very few calories, and if my carbohydrate intake goes up, I gain weight.

In my Facebook groups, I speak openly about the difficulty of staying keto and/or low-carb over a sustained period of time. In my case, "carbohydrate addiction" is not far from the truth. I do crave carbs. (Yes, I do understand it may not be a scientific construct, but behaviorally, for all intents and purposes, I have been known to act as though I am addicted. One cupcake is not enough, and one cupcake is also one too many.)

I have to be ever-vigilant. I have to stay on guard. I have to accept that it will take me a month to lose what I gain in a week of indulgence. It is frustrating, it is unfair—but that is my reality.

Does all this sound familiar to you? Have you had similar struggles, a similar story, a similar path toward keto? Are you still struggling with the unfairness of it all?

Let's talk about that unfairness.

WEIGHT GAIN AND ANGER

I don't see people speaking about this openly, but I am sure that I am not the only one who has experienced this. When surrounded by thin people who seemingly eat whatever they want and stay skinny, while you watch every calorie that goes into your mouth, it's difficult not to be angry, not to rail at the universe, not to have a little pity party about how unfair things are and how unlucky you are to gain weight so easily.

I will admit that there were times it was difficult for me to even think about what to do to lose weight, because thinking about it would fill me with anger. Why was I so unlucky? Why was my metabolism so efficient that it was apparently able to survive and even thrive on starvation-level calories? This was patently unfair and I just absolutely did not deserve this fate.

I know, I know. We tell our children the world is not fair. You'd think we'd know better. The fact is, our heads might know better, but internalizing that in our hearts is not the same thing.

This continued for years, which is both ridiculous and shameful really: a grown woman railing against the unfairness in the world for being overweight. Then one day, I realized that if I were going to complain about fairness, perhaps I could also complain about all the unfair advantages that have been afforded to me. Clearly I won the "lottery of the womb" when I was born into an educated, intelligent, nurturing, middle-class family. Clearly I had had many lucky breaks come my way, in my personal life, in my career, in my choices of friends, in a thousand different facets of my life. Somehow I never complained about the inherent unfairness of luck—just about the one thing in which I had not, in fact, won the genetic lottery! Yeah, way to be overprivileged and ignorant about it, Urvashi. This changed my attitude and mentally prepared me to put aside the matter of fairness (or lack thereof) and focus on what I could do, rather than on why I should not have to do anything at all in the first place.

I mention all this because in conversations with others I realized that this is a deterrent for many of us. The sheer unfairness, the refusal to accept that some of us just need to make more radical changes than others in order to lose weight, the belief that we should be able to eat like others and have our bodies deal with foods like others seem to—all these things keep us from accepting the truth and moving on to doing what is needed.

If you are struggling with these thought patterns and issues, I recommend that part of your recovery and the foundation for the dietary change you need to make in your life will need to involve acceptance of your metabolism. Without this acceptance, you will be tempted to "eat like other people," to believe you can do what others do, to think it's unfair and therefore that you should not have to change.

Know that you are not alone. For many of us, what is needed is strict control over carbohydrates. Many of us gain weight on not much food, especially if it's the wrong type of food. Many of us absolutely cannot and should not be eating five times a day. Many of us do not lose fifty pounds in three months. Many of us stall for weeks on end, even though we are doing the right things. If you are one of those people, you are one of my tribe. You and I may have to eat differently, eat less often, fast for long periods of time, and monitor our intake carefully—for the rest of our lives.

So let's talk about what needs doing to lose this weight, and/or to keep it off. The first thing that is required is a better understanding of why we gain weight.

UNDERSTANDING THE MECHANICS OF WEIGHT LOSS

I like to understand why things work as they do. Simply giving me rules just doesn't work for me. In fact, I'm so terrible at following rules that telling me the rule is a surefire way to make me tune out or blatantly disobey you. But tell me why, and I'm a happy, nerdy scientist at that point. Basically I'll listen to science before I will listen to what your neighbor told you or what you think is true.

Let me tell you what I wish someone had told me about the mechanics of weight loss, if you are overweight due to carbohydrate/insulin disturbances.

Here they are:

1. Your body is either releasing insulin or it is not.
2. If it's releasing insulin, you're not burning fat.
3. If you fast or eat foods that don't cause you to release insulin, you will probably burn fat.

That's all I needed to know, rather than all the "eat this, don't eat that, eat carbs only during a full moon while facing west" stuff that I was busy memorizing and trying to live by. Everything else about weight loss and the ketogenic diet focuses on the details of how to keep your insulin levels low.

- You restrict carbs because carbs cause you to release insulin.
- You eat moderate amounts of protein because excess protein can cause you to release insulin.
- You eat more fat because fat does not cause you to release insulin.
- You pair the ketogenic diet with intermittent fasting and/or no grazing between meals to reduce insulin secretion and increase insulin sensitivity.

THIS IS THE BIG PICTURE.

KETO BASICS

The ketogenic (keto) diet is based on a normal metabolic process called *ketosis*, which happens when your body does not have enough glucose for energy and therefore burns fat instead. During ketosis, chemical molecules called ketones are produced in the liver when fat is burned, and they are sent into your bloodstream to be used as fuel for the brain, muscles, and tissues.

Ketosis is probably what allowed our ancestors to survive when carbohydrates were not readily available for long stretches of time. A keto diet reduces carbohydrate intake to encourage the body to burn fat instead.

MACRONUTRIENTS

The keto diet is a low-carb, moderate-protein, high-fat plan, which usually breaks down into the following percentages daily:

- 60 to 75 percent of calories from fat
- 15 to 30 percent of calories from protein
- 5 to 10 percent of calories from carbs

Every single meal does not have to be in perfect balance, but the proportions of macronutrients—carbohydrates, protein, and fat, or your "macros"—should be close to these percentages at the end of the day.

SETTING THE RIGHT MACROS FOR YOU

Everyone has unique keto macronutrient proportions to produce the desired effects (such as weight loss or maintenance), depending on height, weight, goals, exercise level, and body fat percentage. This is why using an online keto calculator can be very effective for figuring out your individual dietary needs. These calculators can calculate your macro numbers and daily calorie count to keep you in the state of ketosis, or get you there initially.

Since carbohydrates (glucose) are the usual primary fuel source for the body, it is important to stay within the recommended macro range when considering your food choices. If your carbs are too high, you will not reach ketosis at all. Some people go into ketosis with 20 grams of carbs daily, while other lucky folks seem to be able to get there with twice as many carbs. The right level of carbs for ketosis and health definitely seems to fluctuate for people, but with a little experimenting, you will find your own sweet spot for weight loss/maintenance and good health.

After a lot of experimenting, I know what works for me. I started the journey at 5 feet 5 inches tall and 230 pounds. My goal weight was 152 pounds, which I reached over 10 interminable, difficult months. To achieve weight loss, I had to eat less than 800 calories per day and keep carbs between 20 and 25 grams. For maintenance, I can eat 1,200 to 1,300 calories per day and keep carbs between 50 and 75 grams. I still gain when I routinely consume 80 grams of carbs or more per day.

To lose a small regain in weight now, I have to fast intermittently every other day and restrict carbs to 20 to 30 grams per day until the gain is gone. Knowing this has helped me maintain my weight over the past 5 years. Clearly what works for me may not work for you, but if you track your intake carefully, you will soon know what is best for you.

I taught myself how to follow the keto diet by consulting three sources:

- *The Obesity Code* by Jason Fung
- *Why We Get Fat: And What to Do About It* by Gary Taubes
- *The Art and Science of Low Carbohydrate Living* by Jeff S. Volek and Stephen D. Phinney

These sources provide the scientific rationale and research that underlie their recommendations, which I appreciate and you may, too.

KETO MYTHS

There are as many myths about keto as there are adherents to the diet. Some may see what I write below as a myth as well, but I want to share my perspective, so you understand how I approached this book and my recipes.

MYTH #1: KETO AND LOW-CARB ARE ENTIRELY DIFFERENT THINGS

These diets may be somewhat different, mainly with respect to whether or not they specify a per-day carb cap. The keto diet generally requires you to stay at or below 20 to 50 grams of net carbs per day. Low-carb diets simply exhort you to eat fewer carbs. Often, the standard American diet (SAD) is used as a yardstick. Average consumption of carbohydrates is estimated at 300 grams daily for most Americans. As you can see, there's a lot of room between 20 grams and 300 grams to specify what constitutes low-carb. Keto and non-specific low-carb diets are similar in that they typically emphasize consuming lower amounts of carbohydrates, similar amounts of proteins, and higher quantities of fat than are consumed in the SAD.

MYTH #2: CERTAIN INGREDIENTS ARE SIMPLY NOT "ALLOWED" ON KETO

Religion, politics, and keto diet rules—these are the known controversies we all avoid discussing with others, aren't they? Here's my approach to keto: I completely exclude excessively high glycemic index foods such as pasta, rice, potatoes, bread, flour, and sugar. These foods are known to spike blood sugar and insulin for absolutely everyone.

I advocate not eating sugar, not even in small quantities. Sugar causes a spike in insulin and often results in cravings for more sugar that can derail a well-progressing keto dieter.

Other than that, I eat real food, and I watch macros carefully. What matters to me is that the overall carb count remains low, and that what carbs I do ingest are from foods that are not known to spike insulin levels (such as vegetables, berries, etc.).

I also count net carbs, which is total carbs, minus fiber, minus sugar alcohols. If you're on a keto diet for health reasons, you should do what your doctor tells you. Me, I'm the wrong kind of doctor to give you advice on that. (If you have issues with your experimental design or statistical significance, however, I'm your girl.)

MYTH #3: EATING KETO MEANS I HAVE TO EAT ALL THE FAT GRAMS MY CALCULATOR SPECIFIES

Most experts agree that we should eat only as much fat as is needed for satiety, especially if you are trying to lose weight. Your goal is to get your body to burn stored fat. This is much harder than burning the fat you eat, which is more readily available for fuel. So your highly efficient body is going to burn the fat you eat for fuel before it starts tapping into your stored reserves. If you keep eating more fat than your body needs to burn for fuel, not only will you not lose fat, but you could gain some fat, which is not what you're going for. The main reason fat makes up such a high proportion of keto diets is because it does not raise insulin. If you're hungry, fat not only satiates quickly, but it does so without raising insulin secretion.

What works for me is to treat protein as a level I have to hit, carbs as a level I cannot exceed, and then fat to satiate my hunger—and you know, because it tastes so good!

MYTH #4: CALORIES DON'T MATTER

Sadly, calories do still matter, for the most part. The type of calories you eat (those from carbs versus protein versus fat) matters quite a lot. We all know that 100 calories of broccoli has a very different impact on your blood sugar and insulin than 100 calories of sugar.

But having said that, it is simply not possible to lose weight while eating many more calories than your body can burn. Keto allows me to eat more calories and yet not gain weight than I can on a high-carb diet. But if you eat 4,000 calories in a day, and your basal metabolic rate (BMR, or the number of calories needed for your body to perform basic, life-sustaining functions, like you know, breathing, processing food, etc.) is only 2,000 calories, it's only a matter of time before you will be shopping for new pants.

MYTH #5: HIGHER LEVELS OF KETOSIS FOR THE WIN!

Higher levels of ketones do not cause greater fat loss. Being in ketosis is much more important than the level of that ketosis. While it's fun to pee on the keto screening strips and brag about the various colors your strips turn, recognize this for what it is—fun and games. As long as you are in ketosis, you are burning fat.

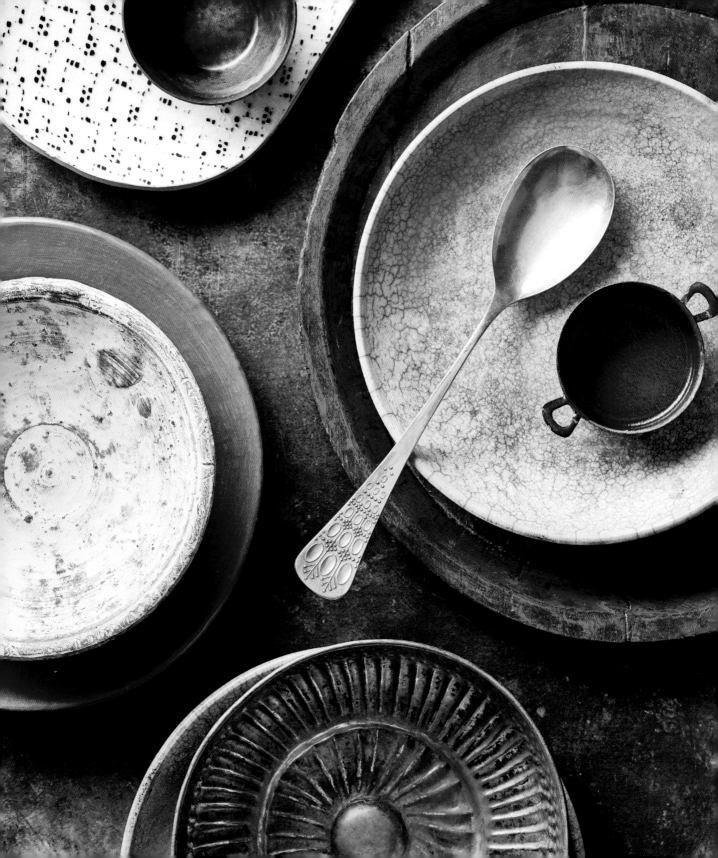

A 4-WEEK PLAN FOR EASING INTO KETO

When my boys were little, I taught them both to read. Mark was reading by the time he was two and a half years old, and Alex by the time he was three and a half. (I wasn't able to stay home with him, so it took us a little longer.) I taught them using a series called Bob Books. The principle of the books is that they start with two consonants and a vowel, and an entire book is written with just those three sounds. Book 2 adds a few additional sounds, and this continues with additional books until the boys were reading effortlessly.

This build-on-it pedagogical approach made it so easy for the boys to keep reading and to keep learning. I also saw the sense of pride they had in reading a whole book by themselves. It reemphasized for me the need for us all to experience small victories as we build a feeling of self-efficacy while learning a new skill.

Weight loss is a long, drawn-out process. If your only milestone is that you will celebrate when you reach a 50-pound loss, you will be waiting for a long while, and you may get a little discouraged. Instead, I am a firm believer in celebrating NSVs, or non-scale victories.

NSVs include fitting into smaller clothes even though the scale hasn't moved. Going for a long walk, turning down your favorite pasta, feeling better than you have in years, joints that aren't swollen—all these are great and delightful NSVs that you can focus on. These are important because much of weight loss, especially the pace of weight loss, is often something you can't dictate as much as you'd like to.

WHAT YOU CAN AND CAN'T CONTROL

I want you to listen to me carefully on this. You cannot fully control how fast your body wants to lose weight. You can only control what you put in your mouth—or don't put in your mouth.

If you're anything like me and a thousand other slow losers, you could do everything you're meant to—and stall, lose one week but not other weeks, lose more slowly than other people, and otherwise get utterly discouraged.

Your body has its own rhythm, its own rate of weight loss. You can control what you eat or don't eat. You cannot dictate to your body how fast it should lose weight.

So I have to judge my success not just on the scale, but in behavioral changes. As a cognitive psychologist, I am a huge proponent of behavioral therapy as a way to achieve sustainable behavioral change. Change your behavior, change your eating habits, change what you eat and when you eat, and health and weight loss will follow. This chapter focuses on how to make these behavioral changes in a manner that is sustainable, gentle, and effective.

Before you start, I should mention something: I am not a medical or healthcare professional, so you definitely want to consult what my sons call "a real doctor, not a PhD like my mom." My only objective here is to show people how easy it can be to start on keto using baby steps and achievable goals.

EASING INTO KETO

Some of us want to jump straight into keto, while others are better off easing into it slowly. We worry that we will start something we won't be able to keep up with, and we use that as an excuse to never start.

If you are someone who prefers easing into keto, I want to share with you the plan that thousands of people have followed, with great success, within my TwoSleevers Facebook keto group. It is a gentle, but effective way to change around your eating habits. Many have also used it successfully to bring reluctant family members on board.

Each week, I will give you three or four things that you will want to do. By the end of four weeks, you will be eating almost entirely keto, and tracking your macros to ensure that you are on track.

I know these tips look ridiculously simple—but they work. There are volumes written on eat this, not that, do this or that, don't eat this particular food unless it's a full moon—but really, there's no need to complicate things that much.

#trustUrvashi, as we say in my Facebook groups. Follow these tips and you will be on your way to good health.

WEEK 1 TIPS

1. **Don't eat:** This week, don't eat potatoes, pasta, bread, rice, grains, beans, and sugar, and limit fruits to two per day.
2. **Do eat:** Eat whatever you want for meats, eggs, vegetables, cheese, nuts, avocados, and fats. Eat meat, nuts, and cheese for snacks between meals if you get hungry.
3. **Find recipes:** Go to my website TwoSleevers .com and find the 170+ keto, low-carb recipes, then choose a few that look tasty to you. Make two or three of those recipes this

week so you can see how you can eat real food on keto. Eat as much as you want of those.

That's it for week 1. Seriously, that's it. No counting, no tracking, no worrying. Just do this all week and you'll be ready to take on week 2.

WEEK 2 TIPS

Keep doing:

- You should already have given up grains, legumes/beans, and pasta/rice/potatoes.
- Enjoy your meat, veggies, nuts, cheese, cream, bacon, avocados, and other yummies as before.
- Find a few more keto-friendly recipes made with real food that sound good, and make two or three of them.

For week 2 you have three new goals:

1. Reduce fruit to once a day or better still, cut it out entirely. Cut out regular yogurt. You can use a little full-fat, plain, unsweetened Greek yogurt if you must, but try to replace with a dab of sour cream instead.
2. Start fasting between meals. Go at least 4 hours between meals. Do not eat snacks in between. So you could eat at 8:00 a.m., noon, 4:00 p.m., and 8:00 p.m., as an example. You need to keep insulin down. Eating causes insulin release. Insulin release = no fat burning. If you get super-hungry, first drink water or a sugar-free beverage of choice. If that doesn't work, eat a fat bomb. This book is absolutely full of delicious fat bombs, many of which are no-cook, so finding a tasty fat bomb should not be difficult at all.
3. Hydrate well. Drink at least 64 ounces of liquid daily this week. Use it to hydrate, to fill your stomach in between meals, and to create a habit. Water really does help with fat loss.

That's it for week 2!

WEEK 3 TIPS

Keep doing:

- You should already have given up grains, legumes/beans, and pasta/rice/potatoes.
- Enjoy your meat, veggies, nuts, cheese, cream, bacon, avocados, and other yummies as before.
- Find more keto-friendly recipes made with real food that sound good, and make two or three of them.
- Fast for 4 hours between meals.
- Hydrate well.

For week 3 you have three new goals:

1. Cut out all fruit except a handful of berries once a day. Over time you may be able to eat more, but this is a good start.
2. Try 12-hour fasts. You should already be fasting 4 hours between meals. Now go at least 12 hours between dinner and breakfast, or breakfast and lunch. Do not eat snacks in between. Eating causes insulin release. Insulin release = no fat burning. If you get super-hungry, first drink water or a sugar-free beverage of choice. If that doesn't work, eat a fat bomb. This may sound daunting, but if you fast at night, you'll be asleep for 8 out of the 12 hours anyway, which may make it easier for you.
3. Start tracking your food intake. Find a food tracker you like and start keeping track of your carbs. Some options are MyFitnessPal, Lose It!, and Cronometer. This week, you're not going to worry about balancing macros—simply focus on accurately tracking what you are eating.

WEEK 4 TIPS

Keep doing:

- You should already have given up grains, legumes/beans, and pasta/rice/potatoes.
- Enjoy your meat, veggies, nuts, cheese, cream, bacon, avocados, and other yummies as before.
- Find more keto-friendly recipes made with real food that sound good, and make two or three new ones.
- Fast for 4 hours between meals.
- Hydrate well.
- Track your food using a good food tracker.

For week 4 you have three new goals:

1. Educate yourself on macronutrients and what foods contain carbs, fats, and proteins. "Understanding and Calculating Macros on a Keto Diet" (page TK) should be helpful. Calculate the appropriate macros for you by using the Keto Calculator on my website TwoSleevers.com (search for "Calculating Macros").
2. Plan and track your daily intake to ensure you are staying within the recommended macros. So yes, week 4 is the one where you finally start to track all your food. I know many others recommend starting out by tracking, but it can be absolutely overwhelming at first,

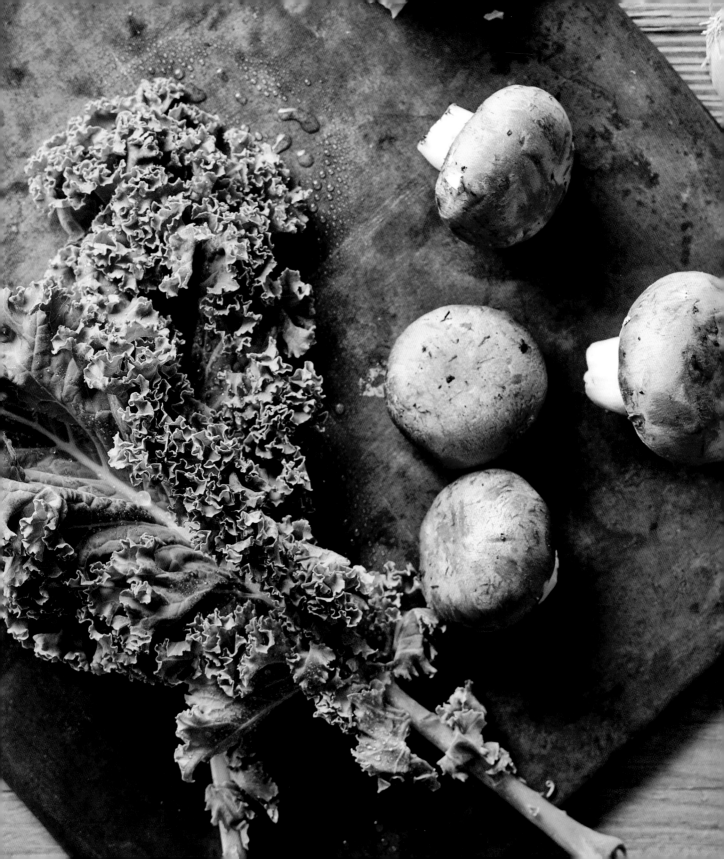

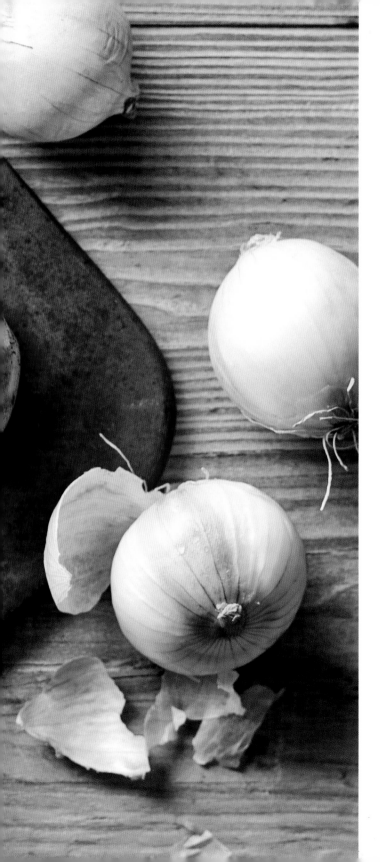

and this is the main reason people hesitate to start keto. So I am asking you to hold off on tracking until you have weeks 1 to 3 under your belt and all is going well.

3. **Try intermittent fasting.** One to three times a week, try to go 14 to 16 hours between meals. Nothing you eat can increase insulin sensitivity or reduce insulin secretion as well as fasting can. Going longer between meals a few times a week can make a huge difference to health and to weight loss.

And that's it. Four weeks into it, you should be eating what you should, not eating when you shouldn't, tracking, losing weight, and feeling better. It really can be this simple.

Do consider joining my Facebook group for support, advice, and camaraderie—all of which can make a big difference when you're struggling. And we all struggle at times, no matter if keto is new or old hat. Finding like-minded people who can relate to your dilemmas can make all the difference on a difficult day.

UNDERSTANDING AND CALCULATING MACROS ON A KETO DIET

It's time for us to get a better understanding of macronutrients and why they matter. My aim here is to be accurate but not comprehensive, so I am going to simplify as best as I can.

Here are the topics we will cover:

- What are macronutrients?
- How many calories are in carbohydrates, proteins, and fat?
- Why do calories matter on a keto diet?
- What are the very basics of weight loss?
- What roles do macros play in insulin release?
- How do I calculate macros on a keto diet?
- What is the difference between total carbs and net carbs?
- Do calories matter on a keto diet?
- Do I have to eat all that fat on a keto diet?
- Do I need to adjust calories as I lose weight on a keto diet?
- What's the bottom line?

WHAT ARE MACRONUTRIENTS?

For our purposes, macros (or macronutrients) are carbohydrates, protein, and fat (C/P/F). Any food can be thought of as a combination of C/P/F. Much of keto is maintaining the desirable balance between these macros, and for Keto Diet Plan week 4 you need to understand this.

In a typical day on a keto diet plan, you want to eat between 20 and 50 grams of carbs, enough protein to maintain muscle mass, and enough fat to provide satiety.

Here's a high-level view of foods that contain a lot of carbs:

- Starches such as pasta, rice, potatoes, bread, and oats
- Sugars such as sugar, honey, molasses, and high fructose corn syrup
- Grains such as quinoa, wheat, amaranth, and millet

- **Beans and legumes** such as kidney beans, chickpeas, and black-eyed peas (but not black soy beans)
- **Fruits,** especially tropical fruits (berries are lower-carb than other fruits)
- **Starchy vegetables** such as peas, corn, sweet potatoes, winter squash, etc.

HOW MANY CALORIES ARE IN CARBOHYDRATES, PROTEINS, AND FAT?

Carbs and protein each have 4 calories per gram. Fat has 9 calories per gram.

WHY DO MACROS MATTER ON A KETO DIET PLAN?

There's a reason you are calculating macros: They serve as a proxy for things that will keep your insulin and blood sugar in check.

People argue endlessly about whether this ingredient or that "is keto." It's not an individual ingredient per se you should worry about—you should worry about being in ketosis. The ways to get into, and stay in, ketosis are:

- Control what you eat.
- Control when and how often you eat.
- Let's talk about what you eat first, and the role macros play in this.

WHAT ARE THE VERY BASICS OF WEIGHT LOSS?

Here is what you need to know about weight loss in a nutshell (assuming your weight gain was related to excess consumption of carbohydrates, insulin resistance, excess appetite, and the like). You are either FEASTING (eating or having eaten within the last 2 to 4 hours) or you are FASTING (haven't eaten in a while). While you are feasting, your body is releasing insulin. While you have insulin in your bloodstream, you are not burning fat.

The way to burn fat is to (a) not eat (i.e., fast) for long periods and (b) eat foods that don't cause you to release excess insulin.

Feasting = Insulin

Insulin = No Fat Burning

Fasting = No Insulin

No Insulin = Fat Burning

Everything else about keto diets is just finding ways to not release excess insulin so your body has a chance to burn fat. As I said earlier, the ways to do that are to (a) control what you eat and (b) control when and how often you eat.

WHAT ROLES DO MACROS PLAY IN INSULIN RELEASE?

Understand these three (oversimplified) facts, and you will understand how to eat for your keto diet plan:

- Carbs will make you release a lot of insulin.
- Protein, if eaten to excess, will make you release some insulin, but if you eat moderate amounts of protein, you will be fine.
- Fat will not cause you to release insulin.

So the way to keep your insulin down? Eat more fat, eat moderate protein, eat very few carbs, and go long periods without eating. That's it. No need to complicate things beyond this.

Let's add that to our previous equations.

Feasting = Insulin

Carbs = Insulin

Excess Protein = Insulin

Insulin = No Fat Burning

Fasting = No Insulin

Fat = No Insulin

Low Carbs = Low Insulin

Moderate Protein = Low Insulin

No Insulin = Fat Burning

As I said earlier, it's an oversimplified view, but accurate nonetheless.

HOW DO I CALCULATE MACROS ON A KETO DIET PLAN?

Let's get this out of the way. There is no magic about the 20 grams of carbs everyone keeps pushing on keto. The right number of carbs is whatever will get you into ketosis and help you stay there. For some people that's 20 grams of carbs. For other people, it's 50 grams of carbs. The majority of us will reach ketosis at 20 grams of carbs if sustained over several days.

There are complicated ways to calculate macros. (And let's face it, I use the complicated ways that involve calculating lean body mass first, etc.) But we are going to keep it stupid simple for our Keto Diet Plan week 4.

- You are going to get 20 grams of carbs.
- You are going to get 60 percent of your calories from fat.
- The rest of your calories will come from protein.

The easiest way to do this is to use a fitness calculator such as Cronometer or MyFitnessPal and let them do the calculations for you. You just specify 20 grams of carbs, 60 percent calories from fat, and the rest from protein.

If you insist on calculating it yourself, follow my logic below. If not, skip to the next section.

Remember that carbs and protein each have 4 calories per gram, and fat has 9 calories per gram.

Total calories: Start out by looking at the total calories you need. I won't repeat those calculations here since there are many reputable calculators out there. Let's say that you need 1,200 calories a day to lose weight.

Carbohydrate calories: We will assume you need 20 grams of carbs to be in ketosis.

20 grams × 4 calories = 80 calories from carbs

This leaves you 1,110 calories to play with.

Fat Calories: 60 percent of your calories will come from fat.

1,200 × 60% (or .6) = 720 calories

720 calories / 9 calories per gram = 80 grams of fat

Protein Calories: The remainder of your calories will come from protein.

I have used up 80 carb calories + 720 fat calories, which leaves me 400 calories for protein.

400 calories / 4 calories per gram = 100 grams of protein

WHAT IS THE DIFFERENCE BETWEEN TOTAL CARBS AND NET CARBS?

Net Carbs = Total Carbs—Fiber—Sugar Alcohols

If you're diabetic, you may need to track total carbs. Many of the rest of us do well tracking net carbs, as fiber and sugar alcohols do not raise blood sugar or insulin levels for most people.

DO CALORIES MATTER ON A KETO DIET PLAN?

Yes, they do. Your body, much like me, is #lazyefficient. Given a choice, it will use energy from food to fuel itself. What you want is to make your body work to use its own body fat to fuel itself. This is a vastly oversimplified description of how your body works, but stay with me for a minute.

The way to make it use body fat to fuel itself is to keep insulin levels low and to not give it so much energy from food that it never needs to, which causes it to use body fat to fuel itself.

So, yes, calories do matter. But two things help. First, you will likely not be that hungry when eating a keto diet because you won't be crashing and burning from carb intake. Second, most people seem to be able to eat more (but not unlimited) calories on keto than on high-carb diets.

I will freely admit research on this is murky, and the usual calories in/calories out equations are not always backed by science. But I have yet to meet anyone who has eaten tons of calories and lost weight. If you can do that, more power to you. The rest of us need to track calories.

DO I HAVE TO EAT ALL THAT FAT ON A KETO DIET PLAN?

Here's what you need to know: Fat grams on keto are a limit, not a level. If you're hungry, eat fat. Remember:

Fat = No insulin secretion = Fat burning.

Personally, I feel that eating protein matters since it helps with maintaining muscle, and when you're losing weight, you do not want to lose muscle. So here's how I treat it:

Protein = Level and Limit. Hit the level and do not exceed the limit.

Carb = Limit. Do not exceed (but you don't have to eat to the limit).

Fat = Limit. Do not exceed (but you don't have to eat to the limit).

So eat fat to satiety. If you're hungry, eat all the fat grams your macros allot you. If you're not hungry, don't.

I eat all my protein. I keep carbs at 20 grams. I eat the fat specified. If I don't lose weight, I cut calories. Since I don't want to cut protein, I have to cut fat calories.

Then this puts my percentages out of whack, and all of a sudden I am consuming less fat as a percentage, and now I want to tear my hair out!

Except. I don't.

Those percentages? Nothing holy about them. They are merely heuristics. What matters is total insulin load and blood sugar swings. Because you know what? If I eat 20 grams of carbs, 100 grams of protein, and whatever fat I need to stay full while staying within my calorie limits, I am. Doing. Just. Fine.

Even if my C/P/F percentages now look like 10/40/50 because I ate less fat that day, everything's okay. Stop worrying so much about details. Focus on the big picture: Keep carbs low. Keep protein moderate. Eat mainly fat to keep yourself full. If you're in ketosis and not losing weight, cut calories.

DO I NEED TO ADJUST MACROS AS I LOSE WEIGHT ON A KETO DIET PLAN?

You will need to adjust calories downward as you lose weight. The easy answer to this is that if you are losing weight, don't worry about re-

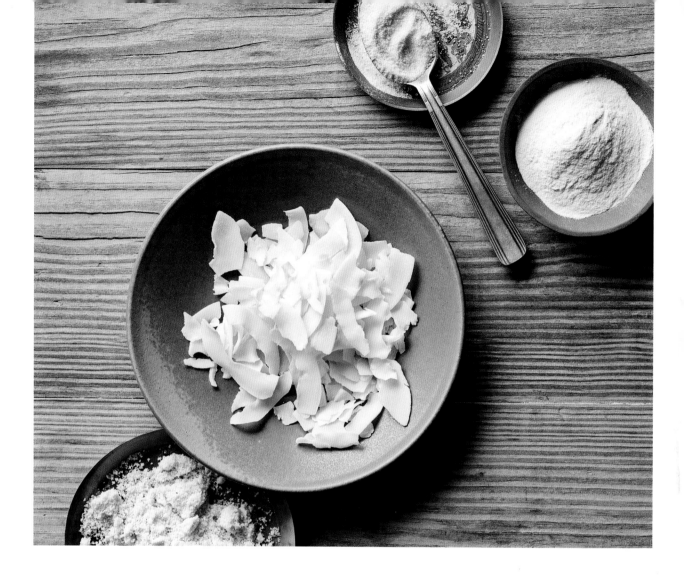

adjusting so much. If you stop losing weight, it's time to tweak.

If you need to be more regimented, then after every 10 pounds or so of weight loss at first, readjust your calories. As you get closer your goal weight, you may have to adjust after every 5 pounds of weight loss. As you adjust calories, readjust your macros.

WHAT'S THE BOTTOM LINE?

Stop worrying so much about details. Again: Focus on the big picture. Keep carbs low. Keep protein moderate. Eat mainly fat to keep yourself full. If you're in ketosis and not losing weight, cut calories.

GETTING BACK TO KETO BASICS

If you plan to adopt a ketogenic/low-carb way of eating for the rest of your life, there will definitely be times when you will fall off the wagon. In my case, that's usually off the wagon and face-first into cupcakes. For those of us who follow keto for serious health issues, this can be dangerous, and the consequences are beyond my professional ability to discuss, so I won't touch those.

But for those of us who follow keto for weight loss/overall well-being reasons, I think this is not unusual. This happens to the best of us. The difficulty often is that one cupcake leads to another, followed by other high-carb things, and before you know it, you're slowly drifting back to your old, bad-for-you eating habits.

Over the last five years, I've definitely had to take myself in hand and get back on keto or low-carb again. Here are the ten ways in which I ensure that I can get back to keto:

Learn to distinguish real hunger from mouth hunger. We eat for a lot of reasons other than real hunger. You have to discover your own reasons for why you eat. I know I tend to munch if I'm happy or bored, and I am easily bored and often very happy, so that's a problem! I'm a lot less likely to eat mindlessly when stressed, so if I wanted to be skinny, I'd just have to stress myself out a lot, but I've found an easier and healthier way than this.

I've learned to distinguish between real hunger and mouth hunger, where I just want something good-tasting to munch on. I do this by asking myself two questions:

- *Are you hungry enough to eat a piece of dry chicken breast?* (which is the least exciting thing I can think of to eat). If the answer is yes, then I'm really hungry.
- *Are you craving something in particular to eat? Or will you eat just about anything reasonable?* If it's a particular craving, I'm not really hungry, I'm just wanting to munch.

If I'd eat just about anything reasonable, then I'm truly hungry. So when I say, *I need to eat something now,* then I'm really hungry. When I say to myself, *Let's see, what sounds good to eat?* Yeah, not really hungry then.

Go back to preplanning and tracking. There's nothing worse than doing well all day and then discovering that you ate something that had a lot more carbs than you expected—and there goes your well-planned day. It's a lot easier to just plan what you're going to eat, enter it into your tracking app, and ensure that you will be on point if you follow the plan.

I find it also helps me to not have to worry all day about what to eat. It's already planned. I just have to eat it—which I am usually more than happy to do. Most of us have to track carbs and calories while on keto, and preplanning helps with both.

Drink lots of liquids. Often when I think I'm hungry, the hunger goes away if I drink a little bit. In fact, for years I used what I called a "water loading" trick. An hour before I was scheduled to eat, I would drink a large glass of water. You'd be surprised how long you can feel full with a large glass of liquid sloshing about inside you.

Weigh all your food. After you've been doing this for a while, you may think you're pretty good at being able to guesstimate weight, but if you go over an ounce or two at each meal, that adds up to several hundred more calories than you should be eating. I also know that sometimes when I've gone back to weighing my food, I've been eating less than I should have because what I considered a 4-ounce piece of chicken actually turned out to only be 3 ounces. Weighing or measuring out your portions really

helps you stay on track. It also re-introduces a discipline around meals that I may have lost when I fell off the wagon.

Fast between meals. NO grazing. This is critical on keto. Remember, you're trying to reduce insulin and reduce spikes in blood sugar. Nothing reduces insulin secretion as well as fasting. I usually set my clock to 4 hours between meals. If I get hungry within 3 or 4 hours of my last meal, I drink something instead, because it was really unlikely be real hunger. Not only does it limit calories, but it also reduces my insulin response. I have to remember that I am either feasting (eating) or fasting (going without food). And your body doesn't burn fat when feasting, so the longer I fast, the more I burn.

I usually set my clock for mealtimes to be 8:00 a.m., noon, 4:00 p.m., and a snack at 8:00 p.m. This also has the benefit of letting me fast for 12 hours overnight. You may prefer other times, but clock watching at first, when you have been eating at all times of day or night, is a good way to introduce some discipline into your life.

Identify carb levels for weight loss, for weight gain, and for maintenance, and then plan accordingly. In my case, I have to keep carbs below 20 to 40 grams for weight loss, and below 75 grams for maintenance. I am super carb-sensitive. While others can eat a lot more than 75 grams for maintenance (after all, 100 to 150 grams is considered low-carb by American standards), I didn't win the genetic lottery on this one.

You will have to experiment to find the appropriate levels for you, but once you know the levels, it makes planning a lot easier. Typically, I give myself two to three weeks at a particular level of carbs to see if I'm losing, gaining, or maintaining.

Eat more protein. Not eating enough protein is what got me in trouble in the first place. I'm a reluctant carnivore and would rather eat carbs than meat. But that doesn't work for me. I know keto is positioned as fat, fat, fat, and yes, eating fat to satiety is important—but so is protein. I try to get my protein in first and then "fill in around the edges" with fat. I also find that protein fills up my stomach really fast and stays with me for a really long time, so that's another reason I find it helpful to get my protein in daily, not just for overall muscle health but also for weight loss.

Accept hunger and don't think it needs to be fixed immediately. We believe that if we are hungry and don't eat, we will keep getting hungrier and hungrier until we just faint away like a Victorian lady. But most of us do not find that to be the case. Instead, hunger comes and goes in waves.

Often if I am hungry and I drink something or distract myself with something or tell myself I need to wait for two more hours, the hunger goes away. The truth is, there's no way to lose weight without being hungry. Keto makes you less hungry than just restricting calories while continuing to eat carb-laden foods, but most of us have to learn to embrace the hunger. When I feel like I'm starving, I tell myself my body must be burning fat if I'm that ravenous, and that makes it easier to deal with.

Be patient. Rarely, if ever, have I lost more than a pound every other week. Sometimes I've stalled for 6 to 8 weeks.

So if I want to lose 10 pounds—the same 10 pounds that only took a week in Italy to jump onto my body—it could be close to 4 months before I can lose them. It's not fair, but it's my reality, so I just need to get into that medium- to long-term mind-set, rather than expecting miracles each time I get on the scale in the morning. This is easier said than done, I know, especially when the interwebz are full of people telling you how they lost 50 pounds in a month. I hate envy those people. But that is not how it works for me, and that is not how it works for thousands of other silent sufferers.

Allow yourself some treats so you don't feel deprived, but make them keto treats. This is where my book *Keto Fat Bombs, Sweets &*

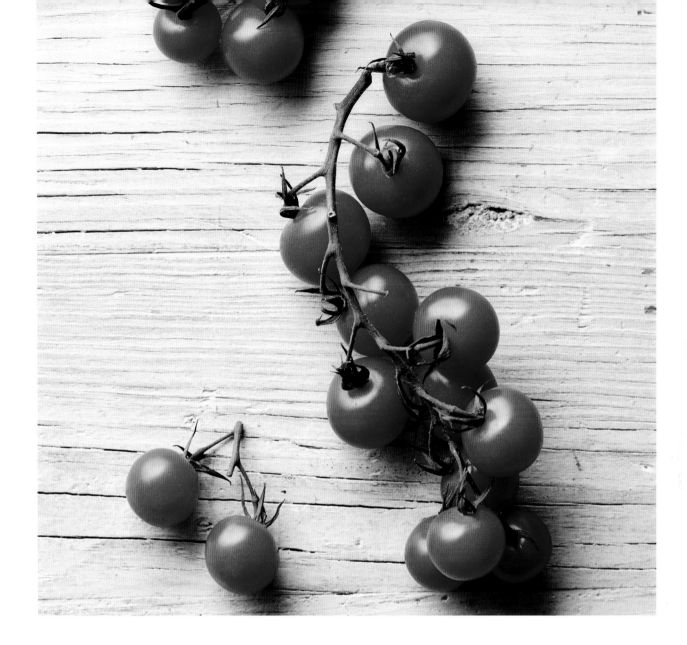

Treats comes in handy. What works for me is to have something planned and ready so that when the craving hits, I can grab a quick little keto treat and not feel deprived. Most of the recipes in this book also serve as fat bombs, so you will be satisfying your taste buds, your hunger, and your macros all in one fell and delicious swoop.

Okay, enough reading! Time to start cooking and eating. I wish you good health, and lovely meals—and lots of guilt-free desserts.

THE RIGHT MIND-SET FOR KETO COOKING

KETO IS ALL BUTTER AND BACON, RIGHT?

Wrong. I don't know why people emphasize butter and bacon over other delicious things. For me, keto is all deliciousness in the form of meat, vegetables, and dairy products. It's just real, healthy, unprocessed food for the most part.

The key to keto for me, is to focus on what I CAN eat, not what I can't eat. An attitude of plenty is a lot better way to live than worrying about what you're losing—and this is true for more than food, as we know!

In this book, I've tried to cover a large variety of meats and vegetables. But I also want you to open up your perception of what constitutes a recipe.

I invite you to think of these recipes as guidelines. Love the Harissa Lamb Chops (page 181)? Why not make chicken harissa another day? Like the Asparagus Mushroom Stir Fry (page 83)? How about substituting broccoli for the asparagus?

You may have to adjust cook times, but the fun you will have in coming up with your own combinations will be well worth the small experiments you will be conducting.

Don't forget to find the Twosleevers keto group on Facebook and brag about your flavorful creations! Everyone wants to hear about them—and I want you to realize all that is possible with cooking.

Don't be intimidated. Many of you know I have absolutely zero formal culinary training. If I can do it, so can you—especially if you start with a fail-proof recipe as your base.

KETO COOKING FOR A FAMILY

Many of my readers struggle at mealtimes since not everyone in the family is following a ketogenic way of eating.

I try to create keto recipes that are just good-tasting recipes that anyone can enjoy.

I would recommend that if you're cooking for your family, you do two things to make this easier on everyone:

1. **Plan for the whole family to share what you eat.** No need to mention that it's keto! It's just meat, veggies, eggs, and dairy.
2. **Make a carby side dish such as potatoes, pasta, bread, or rice for the family.** Sit on the other side of the table, far away from it so you don't "accidentally" have some jump on your plate.

That's it. You do not need to make any other changes to ensure everyone can eat most of the same meal together. There is nothing in these recipes that is "weird." They use natural, whole ingredients for the most part.

The only exceptions might be the desserts that use almond flour and Swerve or Truvía, which while natural ingredients, may not be ingredients non-keto members consume. I can tell you that all the desserts in this book have been non-keto family member approved, thanks to the various testers in my Facebook group that snuck the desserts into their unsuspecting family members.

But the appetizers, entrees, salads, soups etc., are all just plain everyday good food, so plan to share and make mealtimes easier on everyone.

NO-COOK KETO SNACKS

While you should try to limit mindless snacking as a rule, sometimes you just need a snack. Here's a small list of the perfect snacks you can have while on a ketogenic diet.

Best of all? No cooking required.

I get that you're looking for recipes in a cookbook, and I have lots and lots of delicious ones for you! But on the days you just can't even, here are some good choices.

When you're out and about or in between meals and get hungry, impulsive snack choices can be difficult. For me, that's when non-keto, unhealthy choices can start calling my name. In order to avoid making poor choices, I always keep some good keto snacks close by.

For me, what makes a good snack is that it must be easy grab and it has to require very little to no prep, since I do plenty of cooking for meals. Of course follow the keto guidelines of no sugar and low- or no carb with plenty of good fat.

In the sections below I've listed some ideas of low- or no carb foods based on where you can find them in the grocery store. You can bring this list along when you go shopping so you always have snacks on hand for keto snacks on the go, late-night snacks, or a keto-friendly movie snack.

KETO SNACKS AT THE DELI

Deli Meat and Cheese Rollup. One of the quickest and easiest keto snacks. Just make sure that you are buying quality deli meats that don't include fillers, and stay away from honey or maple flavors that add sugar and carbs to the meat.

You can make these as elaborate as you want by adding cream cheese, mayonnaise, lettuce, cucumbers, etc. between the meat and cheese, but when I'm on the go I keep it simple and just wrap a slice of roast beef or salami around a slice of cheese or cheese stick.

Cheese. I will often try different kinds of cheeses from the deli. I chop them into cubes as soon as I get home from the grocery store so they are portable if I need a quick snack to take with me. If you want your cheese to crunch, homemade Cheese Crisps (page 104) are a great way to go.

Olives. Olives really help with the cravings for a salty snack and make me feel full. You can usually find an olive bar in the deli section of your grocery store with many varieties. You can also find individual serving packages in the canned aisle with the regular jars and cans of olives.

Pickles. Never in my life have I eaten as many pickles as since I started keto. Salty, crunchy, tangy, and low-carb. Love them. LOVE them. Don't be afraid to try pickled veggies like pickled okra, pickled mushrooms, or pickled onions.

NO-COOK KETO SNACKS IN THE MIDDLE GROCERY AISLES

Salted nuts. Not all nuts are created equal for the keto diet. The best nuts for keto are macadamias, hazelnuts, and pecans because of their protein and low carb ratio. Stick to the basics and stay away from varieties that are coated in sugar. These are great salty-crunchy snacks for the movies because they're easy to hide in your bag.

Nut Butters. It makes sense that the best nuts for keto make the best nut butter, so at the top of my nut butter list is macadamia, followed by pecan, walnut, hazelnut, and almond. I love peanut butter so I do have that straight off a spoon quite often. You just have to make sure it's not one loaded with sugar and hydrogenated oils, neither of which are good for you.

If you have a nut allergy or are just looking for a change, seed butters are also a good option. These are made from seeds such as ground pumpkin seeds, sesame seeds, sunflower, or hemp, and as long as they don't contain sugar or hydrogenated oils, they are fine for keto snacking.

It is important to note here that with both nuts and nut butter to watch your portion size. The typical portion size for nut butter is only 2 tablespoons and for nuts only 1 ounce. It's very easy to lose track of how much you're eating and throw your macros out of whack.

Canned Sardines. Not one that I would suggest as a handy portable snack—and definitely there is no "sneaking" this into a movie theater undetected!—but if you're okay with the taste, sardines are an excellent choice on keto. One can of sardines has 11 grams of fat, 23 grams of protein, and 0 grams of carbs. Additionally, they're high in Omega 3s, high in B_{12}, and contain 32 percent of your daily requirement of calcium and a whopping 70 percent of your daily requirement of vitamin D.

Beef Jerky. Try to get the grass-fed beef sticks and check the nutrition label. Some of the most popular jerky is made with a sugar-based marinade.

Pork Rinds. Pork rinds are a great salty-crunchy keto-friendly snack option and now come in a variety of flavors. These can be eaten alone or dipped in guacamole for an even tastier treat.

Dark Chocolate. Everyone once in a while if you have a sweet tooth it's okay to indulge in dark chocolate as long as it meets the following criteria:

- The chocolate should have a minimum of 70 percent cacao.
- Each bar should have minimal ingredients.
- Do NOT use chocolate bars with maltitol which has been known to raise blood sugar. Choose stevia- or erythritol-sweetened bars instead.

LOW-CARB SNACKS IN THE DAIRY SECTION

Hard-Boiled Eggs. Hard-boiled eggs are one of the best snacks—they are nutritious, portable, and don't make a mess. I like to pre-peel mine and put a couple in a small container, sprinkled with a little paprika and salt. I love these so much that I have a whole chart on what you can do with hard-cooked eggs in this book (page 114).

String Cheese (as well as other hard cheese cubes). Look for the full-fat versions to keep on hand.

Cheese Crisps. Use your favorite cheese (I like Parmesan) and make my super-simple Cheese Crisps recipe (page 104).

KETO NO-COOK SNACKS IN THE PRODUCE SECTION

Avocados. One of the best keto fats around and easy to simply cut open and eat right out of the shell or perhaps sprinkle some salt and pepper on it. If you have some time, you can make guacamole. This is one of my favorite snacks and I often eat it with just a spoon. You can also buy ready-made, minimally processed guacamole. Look for single-serving portions if you can. These are great because they don't have time to go bad once you open them and they're portion controlled.

Veggie Sticks. Chop up cucumber and celery for a delicious and healthy quick snack. Keep them in the fridge until you are ready to leave or dip in guacamole or a keto dressing if you're staying home.

Berries. If you would like to get a fruit fix you can have raspberries, strawberries, or blackberries in small amounts. Sometimes I freeze them to have a frozen treat and slow down my snacking. 100 grams (about 3 handfuls) have 5 to 6 grams of carbs. See page 46 for a list of low-carb fruits, vegetables, and nuts.

KETO FAT BOMBS

Last but not least: With just a little prep work you can make fat bombs. Fat bombs are a great way to stay in ketosis because they are so high in fat and low in protein that they will help you burn more fat for fuel. You can make many of the fat bombs in *my Keto Fat Bombs, Sweets & Treats* book in bulk and keep them in the fridge or freezer until you're ready to eat them. You can find this on Amazon, Barnes & Noble and wherever books are sold.

It takes so little effort now to plan ahead and have keto-friendly snacks on hand, so you don't make hunger-based bad decisions. And with the snacks I've mentioned, you won't feel like you're missing out on anything!

BEST LOW-CARB FRUITS, VEGETABLES, AND NUTS

The one thing most new low-carbers and those trying to live a keto lifestyle don't often consider is the carb content of other foods such as vegetables, fruits, and nuts. I mean, since they aren't bready foods, that means they're safe, right?

Well, yes-ish. Maybe. Sometimes. Depends.

That's why I've put together this super-convenient guide of the Best Low-Carb Fruits, Vegetables, and Nuts for a Keto way of eating.

It's perfect for sticking on the fridge or carrying with you to the grocery store when shopping for groceries for the week. Trust me, there's nothing worse than getting back home from the grocery store with bags of stuff you *thought* was low-carb only to find out you were sadly mistaken.

NOTE: All of these fruits, vegetables, and nuts have 9 grams of net carbs or less per serving. Most of them have fewer than 3 grams of net carbs per serving.

LOW-CARB FRUITS

It's a common misconception that the sugar from fruits are good for you just because they come from fruits. Sadly, in the world of low-carb and keto, sugar = carbs no matter what the source may be. But don't fret, fruit isn't completely off the menu.

WHAT FRUITS CAN I EAT ON A LOW-CARB DIET?

When it comes to choosing low-carb fruits, berries are your safest bet. Now, just because they're *lower* in carbs doesn't mean you can eat all you want without reserve. They have to be eaten in moderation in order for you not to kick yourself out of ketosis.

There are still quite a few other fruits you can enjoy on a low-carb diet that aren't berries. Plums, coconut, and star fruit are some safe, lower-carb options that you can enjoy as a snack when trying to keep things low-carb.

You'll just want to make sure that you're not exceeding your daily allowance for carb consumption and that you're getting enough fat in your diet in order to get into ketosis.

Though avocados, tomatoes, and olives may not look like fruits, they are actually classified as fruits. And since this is a list of the *best* low-carb fruits, and these fruits happen to have some of the lowest carb content of all the fruit options out there, I decided to include them.

BEST LOW-CARB FRUITS

Avocados (1 cup, sliced)—2 grams net carbs / 10 grams dietary fiber / 12 grams total carbs

Blackberries (1 cup)—6 grams net carbs / 8 grams dietary fiber / 14 grams total carbs

Tomatoes (1 cup, chopped)—4.9 grams net carbs / 2.2 grams dietary fiber / 7.1 grams total carbs

Star Fruit (1 medium fruit 3⅝ inches long)— 3.5 grams net carbs / 2.5 grams dietary fiber / 6 grams total carbs

Raspberries (1 cup)—7 grams net carbs / 8 grams dietary fiber / 15 grams total carbs

Strawberries (1 cup, halves)—9 grams net carbs / 3 grams dietary fiber / 12 grams total carbs

Coconut (⅓ cup)—1.7 grams total carbs / 2.3 grams dietary fiber / 4 grams total carbs

Plum (1 fruit 2⅛ inches in diameter)— 6.6 grams net carbs / 0.9 gram dietary fiber / 7.5 grams total carbs

Blueberries (½ cup)—8.7 grams net carbs / 1.8 grams dietary fiber / 10.5 grams total carbs

Olives (10 average sized green olives)— 0.2 grams net carbs / 1.1 grams dietary fiber / 1.3 grams total carbs

LOW-CARB VEGETABLES

Vegetables are definitely going to be one of your go-to foods for a low-carb diet. They can be used as a side, an appetizer, a snack, or they can even be transformed into something completely different like the delicious Cauliflower Breadsticks recipe (page 84).

Your lowest-carb vegetable options are going to be leafy green vegetables such as lettuce, spinach, and bok choy. Leafy green vegetables can be used to make a wrap in place of bread in a sandwich, or they can be used as a great alternative to otherwise carb-rich ingredients.

The best way to think about low-carb vegetables is in this way: Lowest are leaves. Next are things that grow above the ground. Highest are those that grow below the ground (root vegetables).

BEST LOW-CARB VEGETABLES

Asparagus (½ cup, or approximately 6 whole spears)—1.1 gram net carbs / 1.4 grams dietary fiber / 2.5 grams total carbs

Mushrooms (1 cup raw, white mushrooms)—1.6 grams net carbs / 0.7 grams dietary fiber / 2.3 grams total carbs

Zucchini (1 cup raw, sliced)—2.4 grams net carbs / 1.1 grams dietary fiber / 3.5 total carbs

Spinach (1 cup raw or ½ cup steamed)—0.4 grams net carbs / 0.7 grams dietary fiber / 1.1 total carbs

Bok Choy (1 cup raw, shredded)—0.8 grams net carbs / 0.7 grams dietary fiber / 1.5 grams total carbs

Cauliflower (1 cup raw)—2.9 grams net carbs / 2.1 carbs dietary fiber / 5 grams total carbs

Lettuce (Iceberg, 2 cup, shredded)—1.2 grams net carbs / 0.9 grams dietary fiber / 2.1 grams total carbs

Celery (1 stalk, medium [7½ to 8 inches long])—0.6 grams net carbs / 0.6 grams dietary fiber / 1.2 grams total carbs

Yellow Squash (1 cup, sliced)—2.6 grams net carbs / 1.2 grams dietary fiber / 3.8 grams total carbs

Cucumbers (1 cup chopped cucumber)—3.1 grams net carbs / 0.5 grams dietary fiber / 3.6 grams total carbs

LOW-CARB NUTS

There are few snacks as incredibly convenient as nuts when on a low-carb diet. They're naturally snack-size, easy to carry around in a small disposable zipper lock bag for a quick craving cruncher, have a long shelf life with no need to refrigerate them, and are wonderfully low in carb content.

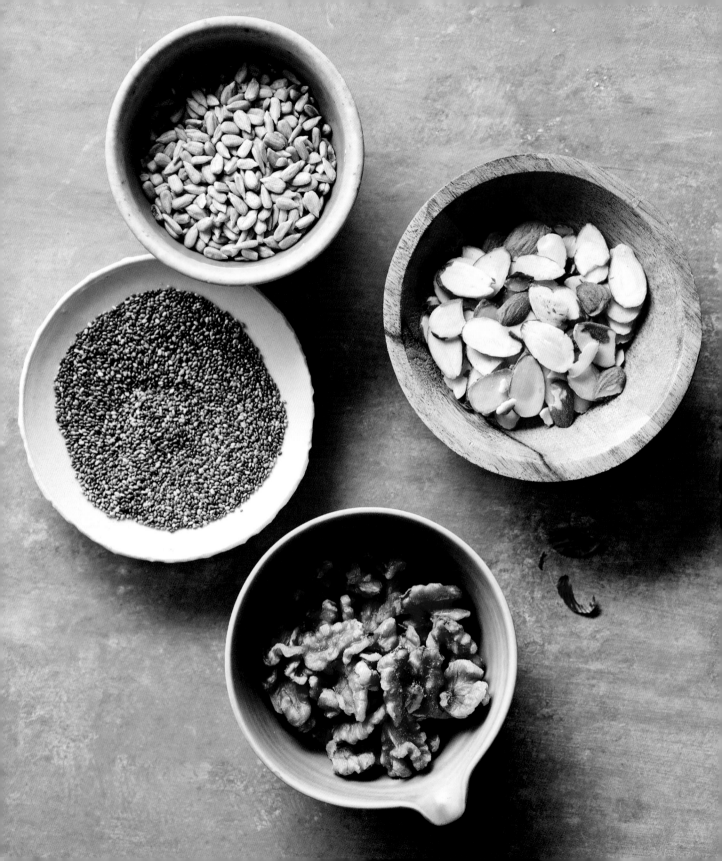

Now, not all nuts are created equal in the world of low-carb foods. Some nuts are exceptionally low-carb, such as pecans, macadamia nuts, and Brazil nuts, all of which have less than 2 net carbs per 1-ounce serving. Others, such as pistachios, cashews, and soy nuts, can be a little higher in carb content and should be eaten in moderation.

Not only can nuts be used as a super-portable, ultraconvenient snack, but they can be used as an alternative to higher-carb ingredients as well. They can be used as a breading substitute to make some of the best breaded chicken you've ever had.

BEST LOW-CARB NUTS

Pecans (1 ounce, or approximately 20 halves)—1 gram net carbs / 3 grams dietary fiber / 4 grams total carbs

Macadamia Nuts (1 ounce, or approximately 11 to 12 macadamia nuts)—1.5 grams net carbs / 2.4 grams dietary fiber / 3.9 grams total carbs

Brazil Nuts (1 ounce, or approximately 6 nuts)—1.4 gram net carbs / 2.1 grams dietary fiber / 3.5 grams total carbs

Walnuts (1 ounce, or approximately 7 whole pieces)—2 grams net carbs / 1.9 grams dietary fiber / 3.9 grams total carbs

Hazelnuts (1 ounce, or approximately 12 nuts)—2 grams net carbs / 2.7 grams dietary fiber / 4.7 grams total carbs

Pine Nuts (1 ounce)—2.7 grams net carbs / 1 gram dietary fiber / 3.7 total carbs

Peanuts (1 ounce, or approximately 28 peanuts)—2.2 grams net carbs / 2.4 grams dietary fiber / 4.6 grams total carbs

Almonds (1 ounce, or approximately 24 shelled almonds)—2.5 grams net carbs / 3.5 grams dietary fiber / 6 grams total carbs

Sunflower Seeds (1 ounce, or ¼ cup)—4 grams net carbs / 3 grams dietary fiber / 7 grams total carbs

Pistachios (1 ounce, or approximately 49 kernels)—5.1 grams net carbs / 2.9 grams dietary fiber / 8 grams total carbs

So there you have it, a comprehensive list of the best low-carb fruits, vegetables, and nuts, also compiled in a convenient chart.

EASY KETO SNACKS

This simple chart of things you can knock together with 2 to 4 ingredients and just a few minutes illustrates how easy keto snacking or cooking can be. Use this as a starting point and make up your own delicious combos.

NAME	EGGS/OTHER PROTEINS	FAT	SEASONINGS/CONDIMENTS
ANCHO CHILE CANDIED BACON	8 slices bacon		2 Tbsp granulated Swerve 1 tsp ancho chile powder
ALMOND BUTTER FAT BOMBS		1 cup almond butter ½ cup coconut flour	½ tsp granulated Stevia
CINNAMON RICOTTA WITH STRAWBERRIES		½ cup whole-milk ricotta	⅛ tsp cinnamon ⅛ tsp granulated Stevia
HAM, CREAM CHEESE, AND PICKLE ROLL-UPS	2 slices deli ham	2 Tbsp chive and onion-flavored cream cheese spread	
CHOCOLATE-PEANUT BUTTER CHEESECAKE BOMBS	¼ cup creamy peanut butter	4 oz cream cheese, softened ½ cup sugar-free chocolate chips, chopped	2 Tbsp granulated Swerve
CURRIED MIXED NUTS	1 cup mixed raw nuts		2 tsp vegetable oil ½ tsp kosher salt 1 tsp curry powder
CHEESE AND CRACKERS		1 wedge spreadable cheese, any flavor 6 100 percent flaxseed crackers	
OLIVE-AND-CHEESE-STUFFED MINI PEPPERS		3 Tbsp cream cheese, softened	

FRUITS/VEGETABLES/HERBS	METHOD
	Combine the sweetener and chile powder. Arrange bacon on a baking rack placed on a rimmed sheet pan. Rub spice mixture over both sides of bacon. Bake in a 400°F oven for 20 minutes or until crispy. Cool. Eat whole or crumble into small pieces.
	Stir together all ingredients. Cover the bowl and freeze for 20 minutes. Roll into 1½-inch balls. Place balls on a parchment-lined rimmed sheet pan. Freeze until firm, about 30 minutes. Store in the refrigerator for up to 2 weeks.
Fresh strawberries	Stir together ricotta, cinnamon, and sweetener. Serve with strawberries for dipping.
2 slender whole dill pickless	Spread 1 Tbsp of the cream cheese on each slice of ham. Place a pickle at one end of each slice of ham. Roll up. Cut each roll into 4 pieces.
	Stir together the cream cheese, peanut butter, and sweetener. Scoop into golf ball-sized balls. Roll in the chocolate chips. Arrange on a parchment-lined sheet pan and freeze for 2 hours or until solid. Store in an airtight container in the freezer.
	Toss together the nuts, oil, salt, and curry powder until nuts are well-coated. Spread on a microwave-safe plate. Microwave on high for 15 seconds. Gently stir. Microwave for an additional 15 seconds or until nuts are golden but not burned. Allow to cool.
	Spread cheese on crackers.
1 Tbsp chopped olives (green or black) 2 mini bell peppers, halved and seeded	Stir together the cream cheese and olives. Stuff into pepper halves.

NAME	EGGS/OTHER PROTEINS	FAT	SEASONINGS/CONDIMENTS
GUACAMOLE-STUFFED MINI PEPPERS		¼ cup guacamole Crumbled feta cheese	
RANCH TUNA SALAD CUPS	1 (2.6-oz) pouch ranch-flavored tuna	1 Tbsp mayonnaise	
BUFFALO TUNA–STUFFED CELERY	1 (2.6-oz) buffalo-flavored tuna	1 Tbsp mayonnaise 1 Tbsp crumbled blue cheese	
ZUCCHINI CHIPS WITH RANCH DRESSING			2 tsp olive oil ½ tsp kosher salt Ranch dressing
PEPPERONI CHIPS WITH MARINARA	6 oz thinly sliced pepperoni		No-sugar-added marinara, warmed
CHILI-SPICED PROSCIUTTO CRISPS	1 (2-oz) package thinly sliced prosciutto		½ tsp chili powder ¼ tsp garlic powder
MATCHA-CHIA PUDDING	1 tsp powdered matcha	¼ cup chia seeds ¾ cup unsweetened Almond milk Whipped cream	2 tsp granulated Swerve
CAJUN-SPICED COTTAGE CHEESE DIP AND VEGGIES		½ cup 4% milkfat cottage cheese	½ tsp Cajun Spice (page 242)
BEEF AND BROCCOLI	2 slices sugar-free air-dried beef	2 tsp mayonnaise	
SPICY SESAME EDAMAME			2 tsp toasted sesame oil Red pepper flakes ½ tsp kosher salt
BROCCOI-CHEDDAR TOTS	1 egg, lightly beaten 2 Tbsp almond flour	2 cups shredded sharp cheddar cheese	Pinch each salt and pepper
BACON -JALAPEÑO POPPERS	1 slice cooked and crumbled bacon	2 Tbsp cream cheese, softened 2 Tbsp finely shredded cheddar cheese	

FRUITS/VEGETABLES/HERBS	METHOD
2 mini bell peppers, halved and seeded	Scoop guacamole into peppers halves. Top with cheese.
1 Tbsp minced celery 2 butter lettuce leaves	Stir together the tuna, mayonnaise, and celery. Scoop into the lettuce leaves.
Celery sticks	Stir together the tuna, mayonnaise, and blue cheese. Spoon into celery sticks.
1 medium zucchini, sliced $\frac{1}{16}$- to $\frac{1}{8}$-inch thick	Toss zucchini slices with olive oil. Arrange on a parchment-lined rimmed sheet pan. Sprinkle with salt. Bake in a 200°F oven for $1\frac{3}{4}$ to 2 hours or until crisp. Allow to cool. Serve with ranch dressing.
	Arrange pepperoni slices on a parchment-lined sheet pan. Bake in a 400°F oven for 5 minutes. Sponge off excess oil with a paper towel. Bake for an additional 1 to 2 minutes. Allow to cool, about 5 minutes. Serve with marinara.
	Arrange prosciutto on a parchment-lined sheet pan. Bake in a 350°F oven until starting to crisp, 10 to 15 minutes. Stir together chili powder and garlic powder. Transfer prosciutto to a wire rack. Sprinkle chips with seasoning. Let cool until crisp.
	Stir together the chia seeds, matcha, almond milk, and sweetener. Divide between 2 serving dishes. Cover and refrigerate for at least 4 hours or overnight. Top with whipped cream.
Raw veggies for dipping (celery sticks, broccoli florets, cauliflower florets, cherry tomatoes, bell pepper strips)	Stir together the cottage cheese and Cajun spice. Serve with veggies.
2 slender broccoli stalks	Brush the broccoli stalks with the mayonnaise. Wrap with air-dried beef.
1 (10-oz) package frozen edamame	Cook edamame according to package directions. Transfer to a bowl. Toss with sesame oil, red pepper flakes, and salt.
2 cups cooked and cooled riced broccoli, squeezed dry	Stir together all ingredients until well-blended. Shape into balls. Bake in a 400°F oven on a parchment-lined rimmed sheet pan for 8 minutes. Turn and bake for an additional 5 to 8 minutes more.
2 jalapeños, seeded and halved	Stir together the cream cheese, cheddar cheese, and bacon. Spoon into jalapeño halves. Bake in a 350°F oven for 10 minutes, or until cheese is melted and lightly browned.

BEST LOW-CARB FRUITS

BLACKBERRIES	serving size: 1 cup	6 g net carbs / 8 g dietary fiber / 14 g total carbs
STRAWBERRIES	serving size: 1 cup, halved	9 g net carbs / 3 g dietary fiber / 12 g total carbs
RASPBERRIES	serving size: 1 cup	7 g net carbs / 8 g dietary fiber / 15 g total carbs
STARFRUIT	serving size: 1 medium (3½" long)	3.5 g net carbs / 2.5 g dietary fiber / 6 g total carbs
COCONUT	serving size: ⅓ cup	1.7 g total carbs / 2.3 g dietary fiber / 4 g total carbs
AVOCADO	serving size: 1 cup, sliced	2 g net carbs / 10 g dietary fiber / 12 g total carbs
OLIVES	serving size: 10 medium	.2 g net carbs / 1.1 g dietary fiber / 1.3 g total carbs
TOMATOES	serving size: 1 cup, chopped	4.9 g net carbs / 2.2 g dietary fiber / 7.1 g total carbs
BLUEBERRIES	serving size: ½ cup	8.7 g net carbs / 1.8 g dietary fiber / 10.5 g total carbs
PLUMS	serving size: 1 medium (2⅛" diameter)	6.6 g net carbs / 0.9 g dietary fiber / 7.5 g total carbs

BEST LOW-CARB VEGETABLES

ASPARAGUS	serving size: ½ cup	1.1 g net carbs / 1.4 g dietary fiber / 2.5 g total carbs
ICEBERG LETTUCE	serving size: 2 cups	1.2 g net carbs / 0.9 g dietary fiber / 2.1 g total carbs
ZUCCHINI	serving size: 1 cup, sliced	2.4 g net carbs / 1.1 g dietary fiber / 3.5 total carbs
CAULIFLOWER	serving size: 1 cup	2.9 g net carbs / 2.1 carbs dietary fiber / 5 g total carbs
SPINACH	serving size: 1 cup (raw)	.4 g net carbs / 0.7 g dietary fiber / 1.1 total carbs

BOK CHOY	serving size: 1 cup, shredded	0.8 g net carbs / 0.7 g dietary fiber / 1.5 g total carbs
WHITE MUSHROOMS	serving size: 1 cup	1.6 g net carbs / 0.7 g dietary fiber / 2.3 g total carbs
CELERY	serving size: 1 stalk (8" long)	.6 g net carbs / .6 g dietary fiber / 1.2 g total carbs
YELLOW (SUMMER) SQUASH	serving size: 1 cup, sliced	2.6 g net carbs / 1.2 g dietary fiber / 3.8 g total carbs
CUCUMBER	serving size: 1 cup, chopped	3.1 g net carbs / 0.5 g dietary fiber / 3.6 g total carbs

BEST LOW-CARB NUTS AND SEEDS

WALNUTS	serving size: 1 ounce	2 g net carbs / 1.9 g dietary fiber / 3.9 g total carbs
SUNFLOWER SEEDS	serving size: ¼ cup	4 g net carbs / 3 g dietary fiber / 7 g total carbs
PISTACHIOS	serving size: 1 ounce	5.1 g net carbs / 2.9 g dietary fiber / 8 g total carbs
PEANUTS	serving size: 1 ounce	2.2 g net carbs / 2.4 g dietary fiber / 4.6 g total carbs
MACADAMIA NUTS	serving size: 1 ounce	1.5 g net carbs / 2.4 g dietary fiber / 3.9 g total carbs
ALMONDS	serving size: 1 ounce	2.5 g net carbs / 3.5 g dietary fiber / 6 g total carbs
BRAZIL NUTS	serving size: 1 ounce	1.4 g net carbs / 2.1 g dietary fiber / 3.5 g total carbs
PINE NUTS	serving size: 1 ounce	2.7 g net carbs / 1 g dietary fiber / 3.7 total carbs
HAZELNUTS	serving size: 1 ounce	2 g net carbs / 2.7 g dietary fiber / 4.7 g total carbs
PECANS	serving size: 1 ounce	1 g net carbs / 3 g dietary fiber / 4 g total carbs

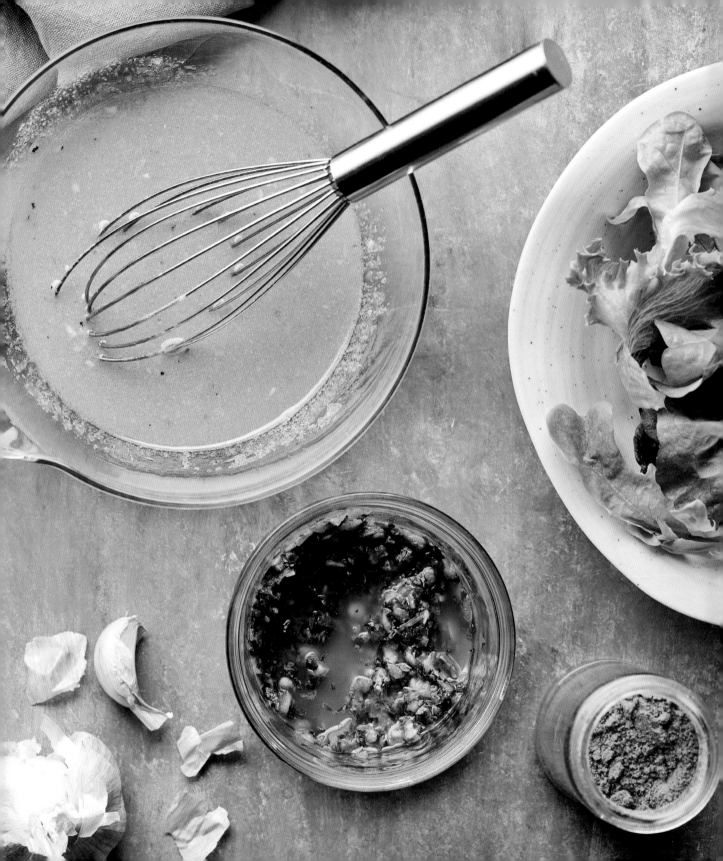

SALADS

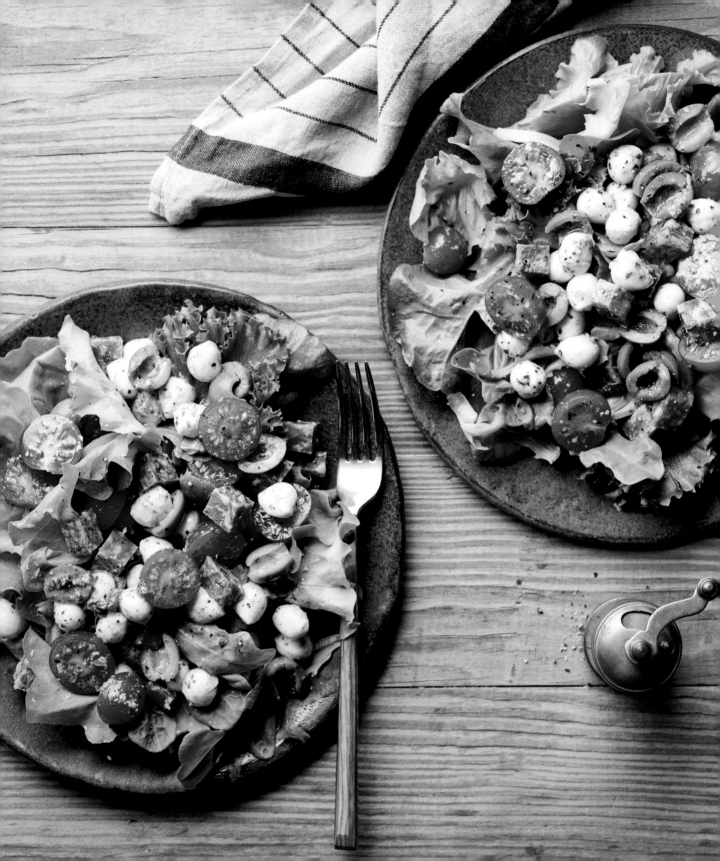

ANTIPASTO SALAD WITH PESTO VINAIGRETTE

Who loves Caprese salad? Me, that's who—and probably also you. Who can eat that much tomato without going over their carbs? Not me, that's who. So, I had to come up with a different way, which meant adding salami, olives, and greens. I don't always have fresh basil at home, so I made this with pesto.

SERVINGS: 4

EGG-FREE
SOY-FREE

PREP TIME:
10 MINUTES

TOTAL TIME:
10 MINUTES

MACROS:

Fat: 74%

Carbs: 6%

Protein: 20%

PER SERVING:

Calories: 278

Total Fat: 23 g

Total Carbs: 4 g

Net Carbs: 1 g

Fiber: 2 g

Sugar: 1 g

Sugar Alcohol: 1 g

Protein: 14 g

FOR THE PESTO VINAIGRETTE

1 tablespoon prepared pesto

1 tablespoon vegetable oil

2 teaspoons apple cider vinegar

1 teaspoon Truvía

½ teaspoon black pepper

FOR THE SALAD

1 cup pearl-style fresh mozzarella cheese, or 1 cup cubed fresh mozzarella

½ cup cherry tomatoes, halved

½ cup sliced green olives

4 ounces diced salami

4 cups mixed greens

FOR THE PESTO VINAIGRETTE: In a small bowl, whisk together the pesto, oil, vinegar, sweetener, and pepper.

FOR THE SALAD: In a large bowl, toss together the cheese, tomatoes, olives, and salami. Pour the pesto vinaigrette over it and mix well.

Divide the greens among four plates. Top each with one-fourth of the tomato and cheese mixture.

VARIATIONS TO TRY

★ Omit the Truvía and apple cider vinegar and use balsamic vinegar instead.

★ Omit the greens and serve in little appetizer cups for a party.

ASIAN CHICKEN SALAD

You can doctor up this salad in a variety of ways—adding chopped boiled eggs, a little cooked ham, smoked turkey from the deli, chopped peanuts or almonds—whatever sounds good that day. For a vegetarian option, you could substitute steamed edamame for the chicken. Sometimes when I'm in a hurry or my hands hurt from my rheumatoid arthritis, I buy preshredded coleslaw mix and make this with that instead. Yummy either way.

SERVINGS: 6

DAIRY-FREE
EGG-FREE

PREP TIME:
10 MINUTES

STAND TIME:
10 MINUTES

TOTAL TIME:
20 MINUTES

4 cups shredded napa cabbage

3 cups shredded rotisserie chicken

2 cups shredded romaine lettuce

¼ cup shredded carrots (optional)

⅓ cup sesame seeds

½ cup minced fresh cilantro

¼ cup chopped fresh basil

1 cup thinly sliced green onions (white and green parts)

½ cup Asian Peanut Sauce (page 233)

IN A LARGE BOWL, combine the cabbage, chicken, lettuce, carrots (if using), sesame seeds, cilantro, basil, and green onions. Toss to combine. Pour the peanut sauce over the salad. Toss to coat; allow to stand for 10 minutes before serving.

MACROS:

Fat: 49%

Carbs: 10%

Protein: 41%

PER SERVING:

Calories: 250

Total Fat: 14 g

Total Carbs: 7 g

Net Carbs: 4 g

Fiber: 3 g

Sugar: 2 g

Sugar Alcohol: 0 g

Protein: 27 g

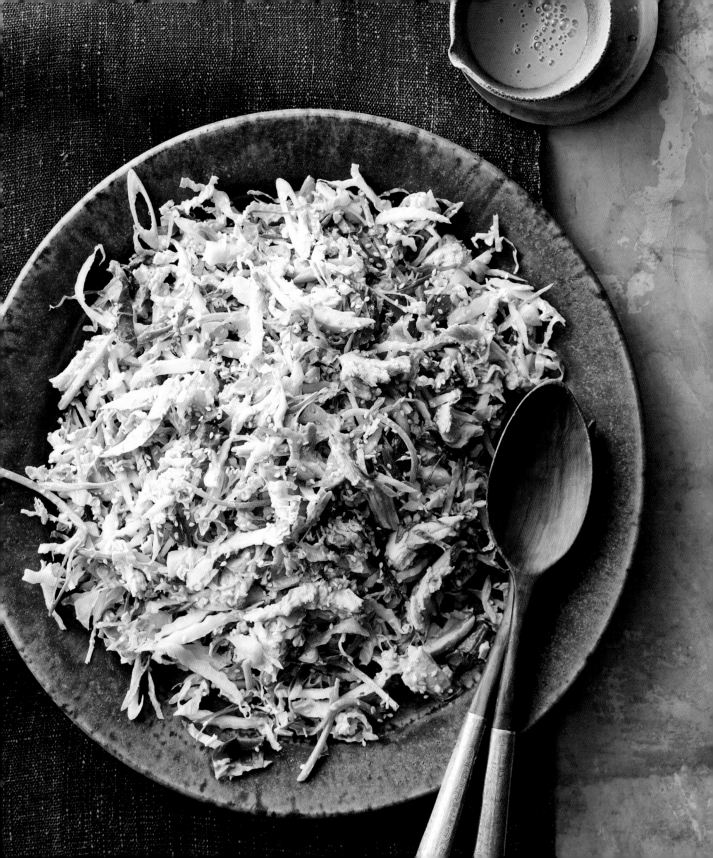

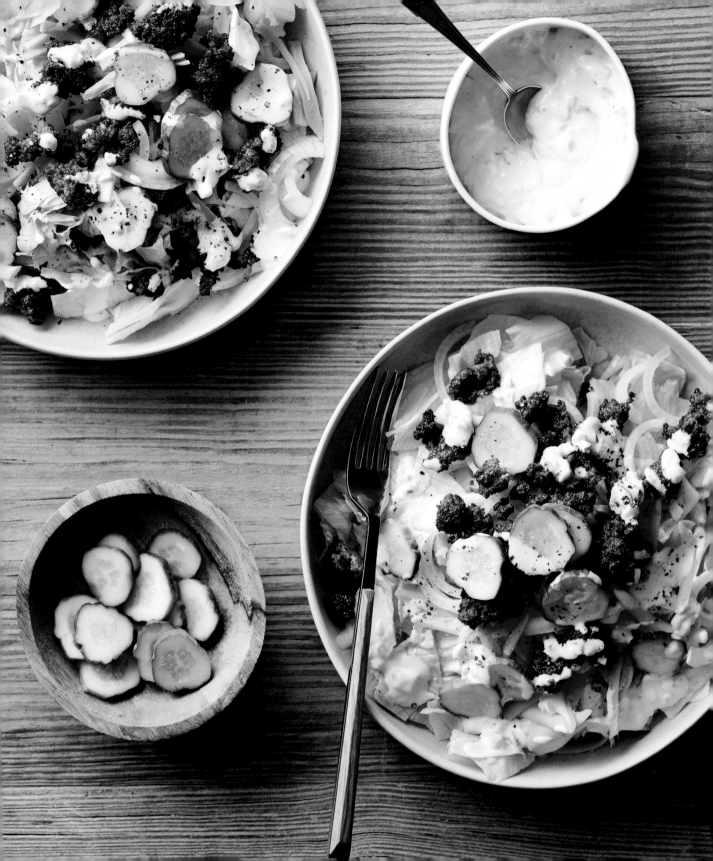

BIG MAC SALAD

I kid you not, this tastes JUST like a Big Mac, except it's low-carb and you know exactly what went into it. My friend Jennifer helped me test this, and she says she ended up eating the dressing just by itself, it was that delicious. Welcome to keto, where you can actually eat a savory fat bomb like a dressing and have that be entirely acceptable—and yummy.

SERVINGS: 4

NUT-FREE
SOY-FREE

PREP TIME:
15 MINUTES

COOK TIME:
7 MINUTES

TOTAL TIME:
22 MINUTES

MACROS:

Fat: 78%

Carbs: 5%

Protein: 16%

PER SERVING:

Calories: 552

Total Fat: 48 g

Total Carbs: 7 g

Net Carbs: 3 g

Fiber: 2 g

Sugar: 3 g

Sugar Alcohol: 2 g

Protein: 23 g

FOR THE SAUCE

¾ cup mayonnaise

2 tablespoons diced dill pickles

4 teaspoons yellow mustard

1 tablespoon white vinegar

1 tablespoon finely minced onion

2 teaspoons Swerve

FOR THE SALAD

1 pound 85 percent lean ground beef

1 teaspoon kosher salt

1 teaspoon black pepper

4 cups chopped iceberg lettuce

½ cup halved and thinly sliced onion

1 cup shredded cheddar cheese

¼ cup chopped dill pickles

FOR THE SAUCE: In a medium bowl, stir together the mayonnaise, pickles, mustard, vinegar, onion, and sweetener. Set aside.

FOR THE SALAD: Heat a large skillet over medium heat. Add the ground beef and cook, breaking it up with a wooden spoon. Cook about 5 minutes, stirring frequently. Add the salt and pepper and cook until no longer pink, about 2 minutes.

In a large bowl, combine the lettuce, onion, cheese, and pickles. Divide the lettuce mixture evenly among four bowls. Top each with one-quarter of the ground beef mixture. Drizzle with the dressing.

> **NOTES**
>
> ★ This would make a fantastic leftover salad as long as you don't mix everything together. Divide the ingredients evenly in four mason jars, layering in the following order: lettuce, cheese, diced pickles, and sauce. Put the ground beef into four smaller microwaveable containers. Heat the beef, add to jar, and shake the concoction like your life depended on it. Voila! Salad!
>
> ★ The sauce will keep for at least a week in the fridge so make a double batch. Great for dipping grilled chicken as well.

CREAMY BROCCOLINI BACON SALAD

I love broccoli salad, but what with the sugar in the dressing, the cranberries and raisins—it's a keto nonstarter. Making my own ensures I know what's in it. I sometimes add cooked ham or chicken to make it a whole meal.

SERVINGS: 4

SOY-FREE

PREP TIME:
15 MINUTES

STAND TIME:
10 MINUTES

TOTAL TIME:
25 MINUTES

MACROS:

Fat: 80%

Carbs: 9%

Protein: 11%

PER SERVING:

Calories: 591

Total Fat: 54 g

Total Carbs: 13 g

Net Carbs: 9 g

Fiber: 4 g

Sugar: 4 g

Sugar Alcohol: 0 g

Protein: 17 g

FOR THE SALAD

6 slices bacon, cooked and crumbled (reserve 1 tablespoon fat for the dressing)

4 cups raw broccoli florets, cut into ¼-inch pieces

1 cup shredded sharp cheddar cheese

½ cup diced red onion

⅓ cup chopped walnuts

¼ cup sunflower seeds

FOR THE DRESSING

½ cup sour cream

½ cup mayonnaise

2 tablespoons apple cider vinegar

1 packet Splenda

1 tablespoon reserved bacon fat

FOR THE SALAD: In a large serving bowl, toss together the bacon, broccoli, cheese, onion, walnuts, and sunflower seeds.

FOR THE DRESSING: In a small bowl, combine the sour cream, mayonnaise, vinegar, sweetener, and the reserved bacon fat. Stir well to combine.

Pour the dressing over the salad; toss to combine. Allow the salad to stand for 10 to 15 minutes before serving.

⏱ EVEN FASTER TIPS

Use precooked bacon. If you're in the habit of using precooked bacon, be sure to reserve some of the fat when you do cook bacon to have on hand for making the dressing and other uses.

Buy the broccoli either precut or from the salad bar.

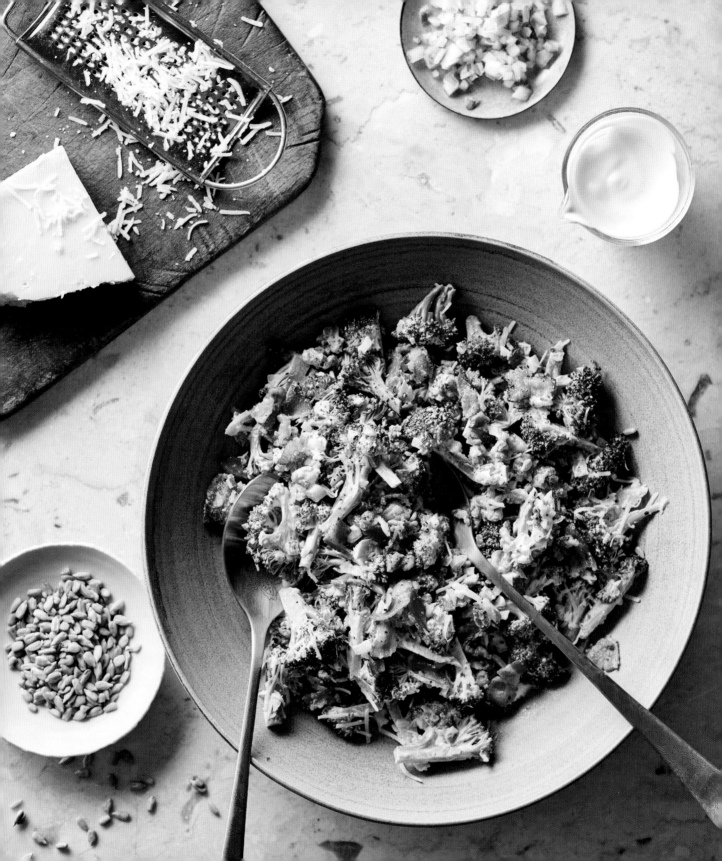

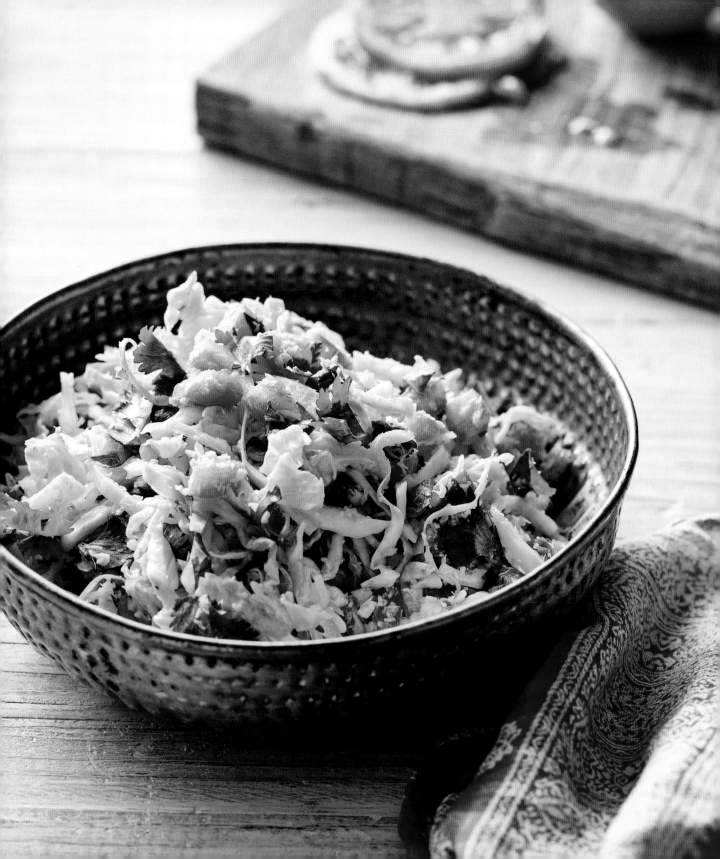

CABBAGE COCONUT SLAW

This recipe is very popular with my readers, and for good reason. If you're not sure about the hot oil step, I have a video on YouTube that shows you how to do that. It's a good, basic, Indian *tadka*, or tempering, and a great skill to have. It's also an excellent way to infuse flavor quickly into oil or ghee. I always buy a bag of coleslaw mix for this so that I can make it quickly.

SERVINGS: 4

DAIRY-FREE
EGG-FREE
SOY-FREE
VEGAN

PREP TIME:
15 MINUTES

COOK TIME:
30 SECONDS

STAND TIME:
5 MINUTES

TOTAL TIME:
20 MINUTES
30 SECONDS

MACROS:

Fat: 62%

Carbs: 29%

Protein: 9%

PER SERVING:

Calories: 102

Total Fat: 8 g

Total Carbs: 8 g

Net Carbs: 5 g

Fiber: 3 g

Sugar: 4 g

Sugar Alcohol: 0 g

Protein: 3 g

¼ cup shredded unsweetened coconut

4 cups shredded green cabbage

1 tomato, diced

¼ cup chopped fresh cilantro

2 tablespoons finely chopped dry-roasted peanuts

1 teaspoon kosher salt

2 teaspoons Swerve (optional)

1 tablespoon vegetable oil, Homemade Ghee (page 239), or ghee

¼ teaspoon black mustard seeds or cumin seeds

½ teaspoon ground turmeric

1 green serrano chile, stemmed and cut into 4 or 5 pieces

Juice of 1 lemon

IN A SMALL BOWL, combine the coconut and ¼ cup water; stir. Set aside and allow to soak for 5 minutes.

Meanwhile, in a large bowl, combine the cabbage, tomato, cilantro, peanuts, salt, and sweetener, if using. Add the soaked coconut to the vegetables.

In the smallest saucepan you have, heat the oil over high heat until shimmering. Add the mustard seeds to the oil. They will sputter, like popcorn, for about 30 seconds. Add the turmeric and chile; stir to combine.

Pour the hot flavored oil over the cabbage mixture; mix well. Drizzle the lemon juice over the mixture. Toss to combine. Let the slaw stand for 5 to 10 minutes. Remove the chile pieces from the slaw before serving.

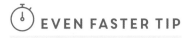 **EVEN FASTER TIP**

Use coleslaw mix to save some prep time.

> **NOTE**
>
> ★ This recipe will keep for up to 3 days in the refrigerator. Over time, the tastes change as the cabbage softens, making it a lovely variation on the first day's slaw.

CEVICHE AVOCADO

I went on a food tour on which the guides showed us how to make ceviche. I was surprised—until a poll revealed that almost no one else on the tour had ever made ceviche. So here we go. Now you don't have to be the person on a food tour who has never made ceviche. Also, I can't tell you how many times I've used store-bought pico de gallo for this. #noshameinthat

SERVINGS: 4

DAIRY-FREE
EGG-FREE
NUT-FREE
SOY-FREE

PREP TIME:
15 MINUTES

STAND TIME:
10 MINUTES

TOTAL TIME:
25 MINUTES

MACROS:

Fat: 60%

Carbs: 22%

Protein: 18%

PER SERVING:

Calories: 303

Total Fat: 22 g

Total Carbs: 18 g

Net Carbs: 8 g

Fiber: 10 g

Sugar: 2 g

Sugar Alcohol: 0 g

Protein: 15 g

12 ounces peeled and deveined shrimp, tail removed, each shrimp cut into three pieces

½ cup fresh lime juice

1 teaspoon kosher salt

½ cup chopped red onion

½ cup chopped tomato

¼ cup chopped fresh cilantro

2 jalapeños, seeded and minced

2 dashes hot sauce (optional)

4 large ripe avocados, halved, pitted, and peeled

EVEN FASTER TIP

Buy prepared pico de gallo and just add the shrimp, lime juice, salt, and hot sauce, if using.

IN A LARGE BOWL, combine the shrimp, lime juice, salt, onion, tomato, cilantro, jalapeños, and hot sauce, if using. Stir to combine. Allow to stand for 10 minutes.

Place 2 avocado halves on each of 4 plates. Divide the shrimp mixture among the avocado halves; serve immediately.

NOTES

★ Make a double batch of the ceviche mixture and store leftovers in the refrigerator. It matures and tastes even better the next day or two.

★ Make a double batch of the tomato, onion, cilantro, and jalapeño mixture (minus the shrimp, hot sauce, lime juice, and only half of the salt). Use as a salsa for cooked white fish or scallops the next day.

CREAMY CHICKEN SALAD

You'll wonder if this salad will be bland and tasteless with just these few ingredients, but I promise you, it won't. It's super-flavorful and extremely easy. But the trick to getting this just right is really that first step where you paddle that chicken but good. That is what gives it that perfect, creamy texture.

4 cups finely shredded cooked chicken breast

⅓ cup mayonnaise

1 cup thinly sliced celery

¼ cup sliced almonds

1 teaspoon kosher salt

1 to 2 teaspoons black pepper

PLACE the chicken in the bowl of a stand mixer fitted with a paddle attachment. Add the mayonnaise. Mix on high speed until mixture is creamy, 2 to 3 minutes.

Remove the bowl from the mixer. Stir in the celery, almonds, salt, and pepper.

SERVINGS: 4

DAIRY-FREE
SOY-FREE

PREP TIME:
10 MINUTES

TOTAL TIME:
10 MINUTES

MACROS:

Fat: 50%

Carbs: 3%

Protein: 47%

PER SERVING:

Calories: 394

Total Fat: 22 g

Total Carbs: 2 g

Net Carbs: 1 g

Fiber: 1 g

Sugar: 1 g

Sugar Alcohol: 0 g

Protein: 45 g

CUCUMBER PEANUT SLAW

Cucumbers and peanuts are probably one of my favorite combinations of things to eat. This slaw—or *koshimbir*, as it is called in India—uses a tempering technique to flavor hot oil. Once you learn how to do this, you can substitute any raw vegetable of your choice in this salad. Just cut the vegetables finely so that the flavor permeates into every little morsel and enjoy.

SERVINGS: 4

DAIRY-FREE
EGG-FREE
SOY-FREE
VEGAN

PREP TIME:
15 MINUTES

COOK TIME:
30 SECONDS

TOTAL TIME:
15 MINUTES
30 SECONDS

MACROS:

Fat: 65%

Carbs: 25%

Protein: 10%

PER SERVING:

Calories: 78

Total Fat: 6 g

Total Carbs: 5 g

Net Carbs: 3 g

Fiber: 2 g

Sugar: 2 g

Sugar Alcohol: 0 g

Protein: 2 g

2 medium cucumbers, peeled, seeded, and finely diced

¼ cup finely chopped fresh cilantro

2 tablespoons finely chopped dry-roasted peanuts

1 teaspoon kosher salt

1 tablespoon vegetable oil, Homemade Ghee (page 239), or ghee

¼ teaspoon black mustard seeds or cumin seeds

½ teaspoon ground turmeric

Juice of 1 lemon

IN A LARGE BOWL, combine the cucumbers, cilantro, peanuts, and salt.

In the smallest saucepan you have, heat the oil over high heat until shimmering. Add the mustard seeds to the oil, shaking to distribute evenly. They will sputter, like popcorn, for about 30 seconds. Add the turmeric; stir to combine.

Pour the hot, flavored oil over the cucumber mixture; mix well. Drizzle the lemon juice over the mixture. Toss to combine; serve immediately.

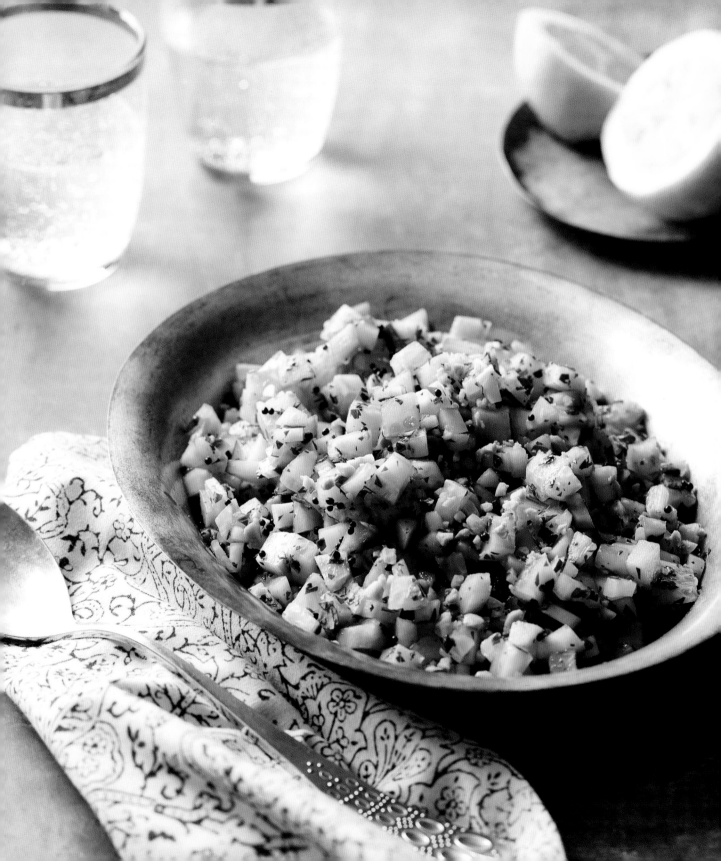

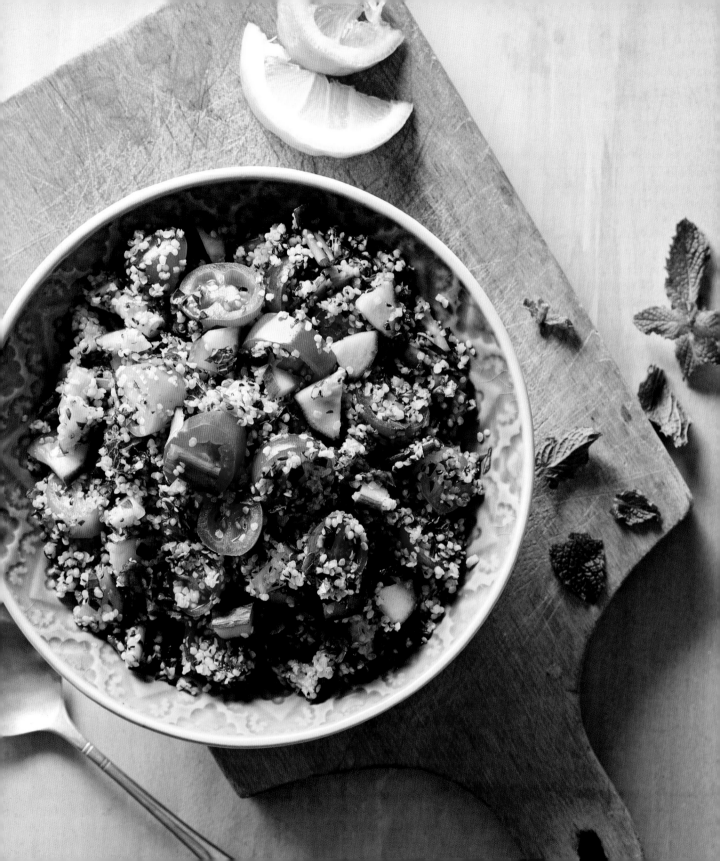

HEMP HEART TABBOULEH

Who needs bulgur when you can have hemp hearts? This easy no-cook recipe gets even tastier as leftovers. What's more, the addition of oil and hemp hearts makes this a great savory fat bomb. For this recipe, you can use whatever low-carb veggies strike your fancy. Any combination of cucumbers, tomatoes, green peppers, green onions, etc. is bound to be tasty.

1 cup shelled hemp hearts

3 tablespoons fresh lemon juice

¼ cup extra-virgin olive oil

1 cup chopped fresh parsley

¼ cup chopped fresh mint

½ cup chopped green onions (white and green parts)

½ cup quartered cherry tomatoes

½ cup diced cucumber

1 teaspoon kosher salt

IN A LARGE BOWL, combine the hemp hearts, lemon juice, olive oil, parsley, mint, green onions, tomatoes, cucumber, and salt. Stir gently to combine.

> **NOTE**
> ★ Double the recipe since this will keep—and keep improving—for 3 to 5 days if kept in the refrigerator.

SERVINGS: 4

DAIRY-FREE
EGG-FREE
NUT-FREE
SOY-FREE
VEGAN

PREP TIME:
15 MINUTES

TOTAL TIME:
15 MINUTES

MACROS:

Fat: 78%

Carbs: 8%

Protein: 14%

PER SERVING:

Calories: 361

Total Fat: 33 g

Total Carbs: 8 g

Net Carbs: 5 g

Fiber: 3 g

Sugar: 2 g

Sugar Alcohol: 0 g

Protein: 14 g

SICHUAN SMASHED CUCUMBERS

There's something very satisfying about smashing those cucumbers with the flat end of your knife. I love how the pieces look sort of irregular, rough, and ready. Smashing allows the cucumber to absorb all the yummy flavors. Once you buy the chili crisp oil, you will find a lot of different uses for it. I often use it with the Naked Wonton Soup (page 187) or just mixed into a chicken broth for sipping.

SERVINGS: 4

DAIRY-FREE
EGG-FREE
VEGAN

PREP TIME:
15 MINUTES

STAND TIME:
15 MINUTES

TOTAL TIME:
30 MINUTES

MACROS:

Fat: 65%

Carbs: 26%

Protein: 9%

PER SERVING:

Calories: 121

Total Fat: 10 g

Total Carbs: 9 g

Net Carbs: 6 g

Fiber: 2 g

Sugar: 3 g

Sugar Alcohol: 1 g

Protein: 3 g

2 medium cucumbers

2 tablespoons Chinkiang black vinegar

1 tablespoon toasted sesame oil

1½ teaspoons spicy chili crisp oil

1 teaspoon Swerve

1 teaspoon kosher salt

¼ to ⅓ cup chopped fresh cilantro

¼ cup roughly chopped dry-roasted peanuts

PEEL THE CUCUMBERS LENGTHWISE, alternating one long peeled strip with one long unpeeled strip. (This creates a kind of "cucumber zebra." This not only adds a little color variation, but also allows the sauce to flavor, but not waterlog, the outside of the cucumber.)

Cut the cucumbers in half lengthwise; use a spoon to scrape out seeds. Cut each half in half lengthwise again. Cut the cucumbers into chunks. Using the flat of a chef's knife or cleaver, roughly smash each piece of cucumber. (You want it to crack but not turn into cucumber purée.) As you smash each piece of cucumber, place it in a large bowl. You should have about 4 cups of smashed cucumber.

In a medium bowl, whisk together the vinegar, sesame oil, chili crisp oil, sweetener, and salt. Pour the sauce over the smashed cucumber; toss to combine. Allow to stand 15 to 20 minutes.

Add the cilantro and chopped peanuts; stir well to combine. Serve immediately.

SPICY KOREAN CUCUMBER SALAD

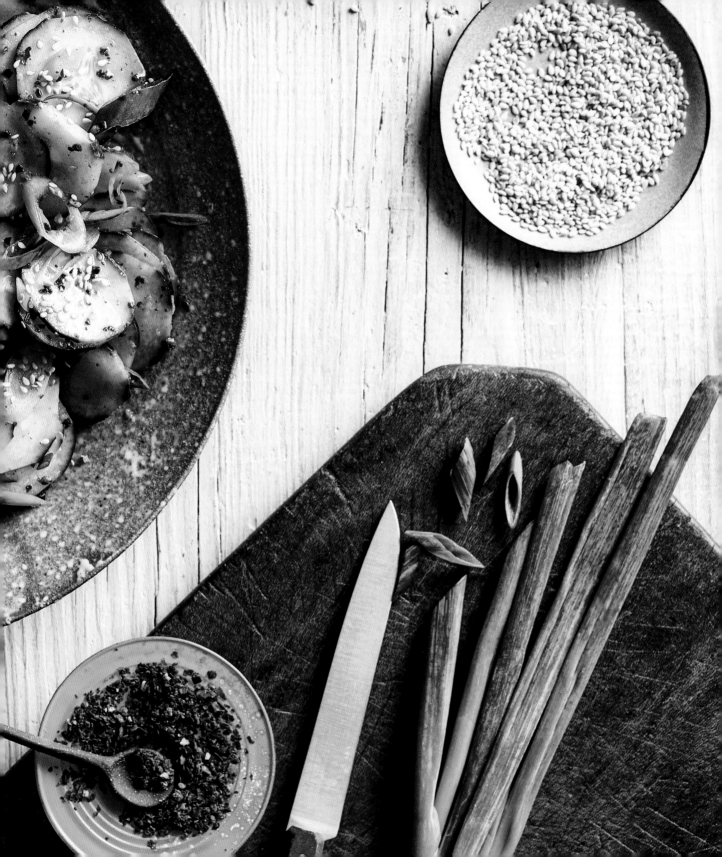

SPICY KOREAN CUCUMBER SALAD

I love cucumber, I love Korean food, I love spicy food, and I love salads. This dish hits it on all cylinders for me. My friend David suggested I try to make this at home, since we totally pig out on it when we go out to eat. What I love about this is that you get two different dishes out of one preparation. In the leftovers eaten the next day the cucumbers have marinated and the result is quite different to eating the fresh salad. Hard to beat a two-for-one dish!

SERVINGS: 4

DAIRY-FREE
EGG-FREE
NUT-FREE
SOY-FREE
VEGAN

PREP TIME:
15 MINUTES

TOTAL TIME:
15 MINUTES

MACROS:

Fat: 67%

Carbs: 27%

Protein: 6%

PER SERVING:

Calories: 106

Total Fat: 8 g

Total Carbs: 7 g

Net Carbs: 6 g

Fiber: 1 g

Sugar: 3 g

Sugar Alcohol: 0 g

Protein: 2 g

FOR THE DRESSING

3 tablespoons white vinegar

2 tablespoons toasted sesame oil

2 tablespoons gochugaru (Korean red chile flakes)

2 teaspoons Swerve (optional)

3 cloves garlic, minced

FOR THE SALAD

2 medium cucumbers

3 green onions, chopped (about ½ cup), white and green parts

1 tablespoon sesame seeds (white, black, or a combination)

FOR THE DRESSING: In a small bowl, whisk together the vinegar, sesame oil, gochugaru, sweetener (if using), and garlic. Set aside.

FOR THE SALAD: Peel the cucumbers lengthwise, alternating one long peeled strip with one long unpeeled strip. (This creates a kind of "cucumber zebra." This not only adds a little color variation, but also allows the sauce to flavor, but not waterlog, the outside of the cucumber.) Thinly slice the cucumbers.

In a medium bowl, combine the cucumbers and green onions. Pour the dressing over the cucumber mixture. Using clean hands, toss to coat, squeezing the cucumbers lightly. Sprinkle with sesame seeds.

⏱ EVEN FASTER TIP

This recipe will last in the refrigerator for up to a week. Over time, the cucumbers get more and more pickled and taste just wonderful.

TANGY SHRIMP SALAD

I've given you a "starter set" for this salad, with ideas for what you can put in it. But really, just add whatever low-carb vegetables you have in the house, and it should be good. The majority of the flavor comes from the dressing and the fresh cilantro (or parsley for the cilantro-haters). If you are allergic to peanuts, use sunflower or pumpkin seeds to provide a little crunch.

SERVINGS: 4

DAIRY-FREE
EGG-FREE

PREP TIME:
10 MINUTES

STAND TIME:
5 MINUTES

TOTAL TIME:
15 MINUTES

MACROS:

Fat: 37%

Carbs: 17%

Protein: 46%

PER SERVING:

Calories: 266

Total Fat: 11 g

Total Carbs: 12 g

Net Carbs: 7 g

Fiber: 3 g

Sugar: 3 g

Sugar Alcohol: 2 g

Protein: 32 g

2 cups mixed greens

½ cup shredded carrots

½ cup chopped dry-roasted peanuts

½ cup thinly sliced green onions (white and green parts)

½ cup thinly sliced raw green beans

½ cup chopped fresh cilantro

¼ cup Tangy Tamarind Vinaigrette (page 237)

1 pound cooked peeled and deveined shrimp (tails removed), or shredded rotisserie chicken

IN A LARGE BOWL, toss together the greens, carrots, peanuts, green onions, green beans, and cilantro.

Pour the vinaigrette over the mixture, crushing the vegetables a little to soften. Add the shrimp and toss again. Let stand for 5 minutes before serving.

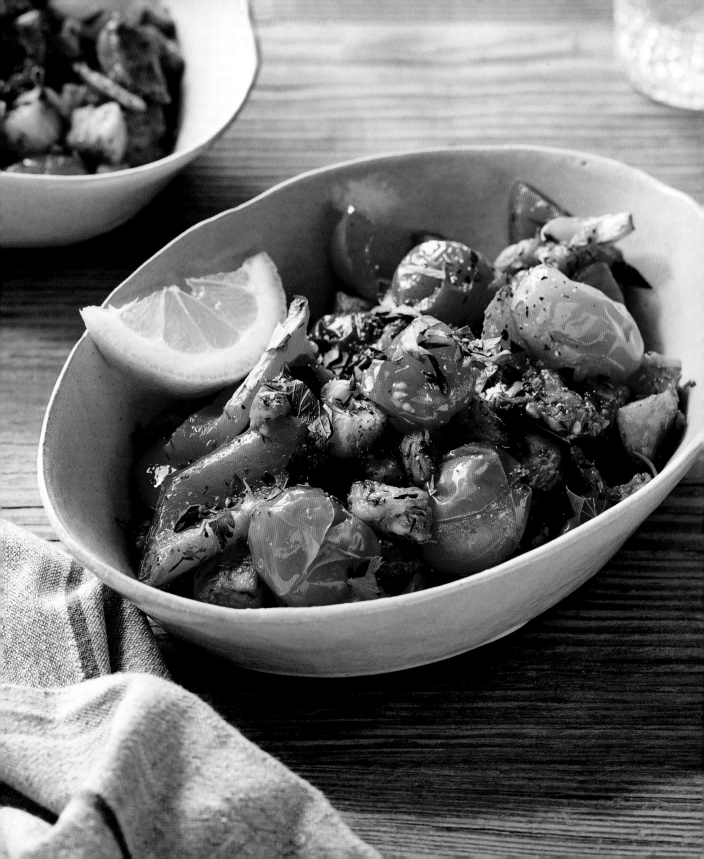

VEGETABLES

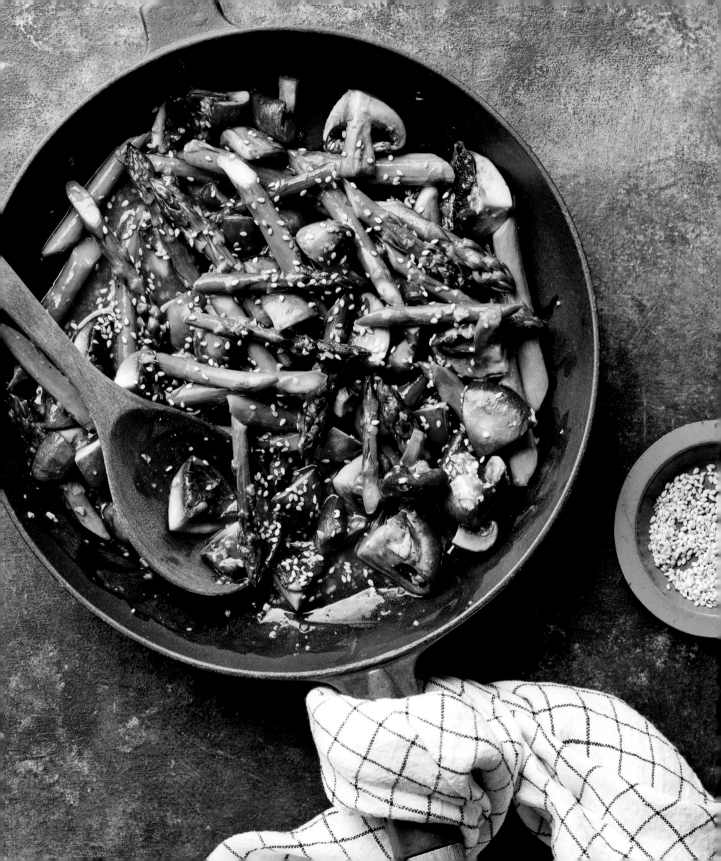

ASPARAGUS MUSHROOM STIR-FRY

To prepare the asparagus, hold a stalk in both hands and snap the end. The stalk will automagically break at the tender point. You're going to use just the tender parts. The Swerve in this recipe sounds odd, but I like the slight hint of sweetness to counterbalance the heat and savory in the sauce.

SERVINGS: 6

DAIRY-FREE
EGG-FREE
NUT-FREE

PREP TIME:
10 MINUTES

COOK TIME:
3 MINUTES

TOTAL TIME:
13 MINUTES

MACROS:

Fat: 53%

Carbs: 33%

Protein: 14%

PER SERVING:

Calories: 67

Total Fat: 5 g

Total Carbs: 7 g

Net Carbs: 4 g

Fiber: 2 g

Sugar: 2 g

Sugar Alcohol: 1 g

Protein: 3 g

FOR THE SAUCE

½ cup low-sodium chicken broth or vegetable broth

1 tablespoon soy sauce

1 tablespoon toasted sesame oil

½ teaspoon sambal oelek or other hot sauce

½ teaspoon kosher salt

2 teaspoons Swerve

¼ teaspoon xanthan gum

FOR THE VEGETABLES

1 tablespoon extra-virgin olive oil

1 tablespoon minced fresh ginger

3 cloves garlic, minced

1 pound asparagus, trimmed and bias-sliced into 2-inch pieces

3 cups cremini mushrooms, trimmed and quartered

2 tablespoons sesame seeds (optional)

FOR THE SAUCE: In a small bowl, whisk together the chicken broth, soy sauce, sesame oil, sambal oelek, salt, sweetener, and xanthan gum. Set aside.

FOR THE VEGETABLES: Heat a large skillet over medium-high heat; add the oil. Once the oil is hot, add the ginger and garlic and stir. Add the asparagus and stir. Cover and cook for 1 minute.

If necessary, add ¼ cup of water to deglaze the skillet. Add the mushrooms and stir to coat.

Pour in the sauce and stir to coat. Cover and cook for 2 minutes.

Sprinkle with sesame seeds, if desired.

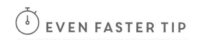 EVEN FASTER TIP

Mix up the sauce ingredients ahead of time and save for 3 to 5 days in the refrigerator. Double the batch of sauce and use it on a variety of vegetables that week.

CAULIFLOWER BREADSTICKS

Yes, I know this takes slightly more than the promised 30 minutes. But this recipe is so good, and such a standby in my house, that I decided to include it anyway. I figured that since I had given you several 20-minute recipes, we'd saved enough time in those to allow me to borrow a few minutes to add to this recipe. Try it, enjoy the ease of not precooking the cauliflower (unlike most other recipes out there), and you'll be happy to wait a few minutes before tucking into these.

2 cups riced cauliflower

½ teaspoon granulated garlic

½ teaspoon black pepper

1 teaspoon Italian seasoning

½ teaspoon kosher salt

1 cup shredded mozzarella or Mexican blend cheese

2 large eggs

¼ cup grated Parmesan cheese

PREHEAT the oven to 350°F. Line a large rimmed sheet pan with parchment paper.

In a blender or food processor, combine the cauliflower, garlic, pepper, Italian seasoning, salt, mozzarella, and eggs. Blend or process on low until everything is well-incorporated and the cauliflower is broken down.

Transfer the cauliflower mixture onto the pan. Pat to an even rectangle about ¼ inch thick. Bake for 30 minutes.

Remove from the oven. Turn the broiler to high. Sprinkle with the Parmesan and broil until the cheese has melted and browned, 2 to 3 minutes.

Cut into 8 breadsticks.

SERVINGS: 8

NUT-FREE
SOY-FREE
VEGETARIAN

PREP TIME:
8 MINUTES

COOK TIME:
32 MINUTES

TOTAL TIME:
40 MINUTES

COOK TEMPERATURE:
350°F/BROIL

MACROS:

Fat: 56%

Carbs: 12%

Protein: 32%

PER SERVING:

Calories: 76

Total Fat: 5 g

Total Carbs: 2 g

Net Carbs: 1 g

Fiber: 1 g

Sugar: 1 g

Sugar Alcohol: 0 g

Protein: 6 g

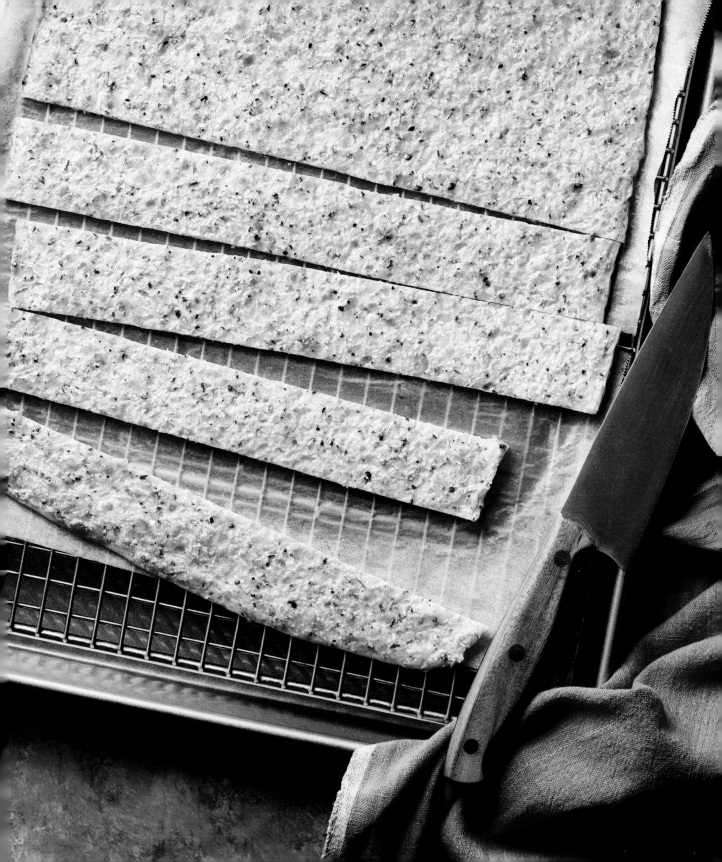

CREAMED SPINACH

Creamed spinach with cream cheese? Absolutely. You know why? Because it's tasty, creamy, and easy, that's why. Leafy greens are so low in carbs, so good for you, so filling—and just plain yummy. If you're not a spinach fan, try it with Swiss chard instead.

Vegetable oil

2 (10-ounce) packages frozen chopped spinach, thawed

8 ounces cream cheese, diced

½ cup chopped onion

3 cloves garlic, minced

1½ teaspoons kosher salt

1½ teaspoons black pepper

1 teaspoon ground nutmeg

½ cup shredded Parmesan cheese

PREHEAT the oven to 375°F. Grease an 8 × 8-inch baking pan with vegetable oil; set aside.

In a large bowl, stir together the spinach, cream cheese, onion, garlic, salt, pepper, and nutmeg. Pour into the prepared pan. Bake, stirring once, for 20 minutes.

Turn the broiler on high. Sprinkle with the Parmesan cheese and broil until the cheese has melted and browned, about 5 minutes.

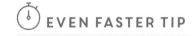 EVEN FASTER TIP

Make a double batch of the spin-ach mixture. For the next meal, stuff portabella mush-room caps (remove the gills) with the spinach mixture and top with cheese. Bake at 375°F for 20 minutes. (Do not stir.) Serve as an appetizer or side dish along with grilled meat.

SERVINGS: 4

EGG-FREE
NUT-FREE
SOY-FREE
VEGETARIAN

PREP TIME:
5 MINUTES

COOK TIME:
25 MINUTES

TOTAL TIME:
30 MINUTES

COOK TEMPERATURE:
375°F/BROIL

MACROS:

Fat: 71%

Carbs: 15%

Protein: 14%

PER SERVING:

Calories: 339

Total Fat: 26 g

Total Carbs: 12 g

Net Carbs: 10 g

Fiber: 2 g

Sugar: 3 g

Sugar Alcohol: 0 g

Protein: 11 g

ETHIOPIAN COLLARD GREENS (GOMEN WOT)

This is a super-simple collard greens recipe. There's not a lot to it but it's simple, tasty, and filling. If you have some Niter Kibbeh (page 238) lying around the house (which, if you don't, you totally should), feel free to add lots of it to the finished dish.

SERVINGS: 4

DAIRY-FREE
EGG-FREE
NUT-FREE
SOY-FREE
VEGAN

PREP TIME:
5 MINUTES

COOK TIME:
17 MINUTES

TOTAL TIME:
22 MINUTES

MACROS:

Fat: 53%

Carbs: 36%

Protein: 11%

PER SERVING:

Calories: 116

Total Fat: 7 g

Total Carbs: 12 g

Net Carbs: 7 g

Fiber: 5 g

Sugar: 2 g

Sugar Alcohol: 0 g

Protein: 4 g

2 tablespoons extra-virgin olive oil, Ethiopian Niter Kibbeh (page 238), or Homemade Ghee (page 239)

1 green bell pepper, stemmed, seeded, and sliced

½ cup chopped onion

3 cloves garlic, minced

1 (14-ounce) package chopped frozen collard greens, thawed (about 4 cups)

2 teaspoons smoked paprika

1 teaspoon ground turmeric

1 teaspoon kosher salt

½ teaspoon ground allspice

1 tablespoon plus 1½ teaspoons red wine vinegar or apple cider vinegar

HEAT a large skillet over medium-high heat; add the oil. Once the oil is hot, add the bell pepper, onion, and garlic. Cook, stirring, until the onions are translucent, 2 to 3 minutes.

Stir in the collard greens, ½ cup water, paprika, turmeric, salt, and allspice. Reduce the heat; cover and cook until the greens are tender, about 15 minutes.

Sprinkle with vinegar and serve warm.

EVEN FASTER TIP

Make a double batch and add some cooked ham for a complete meal the next day.

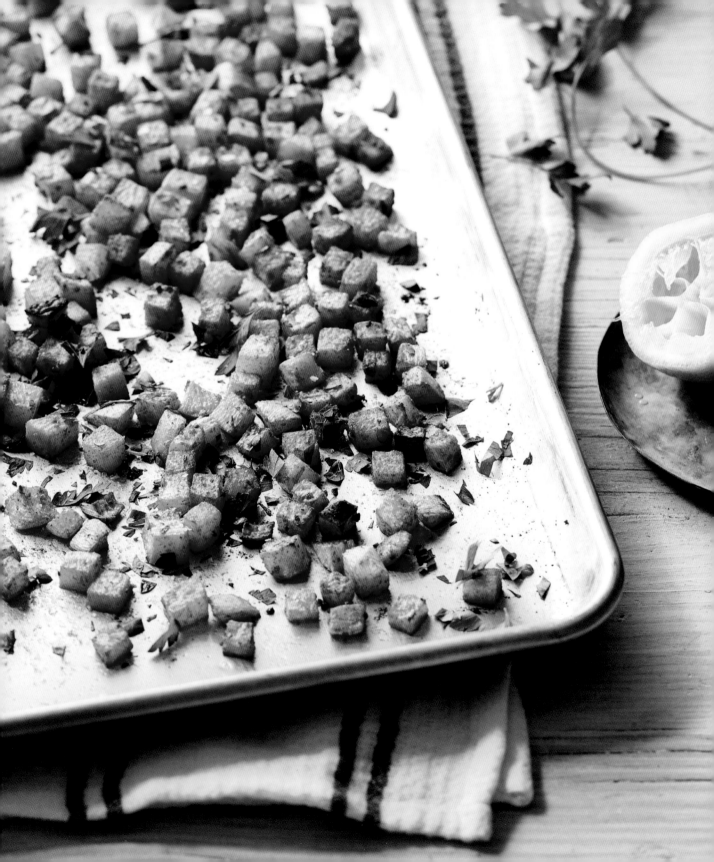

HARISSA-ROASTED TURNIPS

Turnips can take a while to roast. The trick to making this recipe faster is to chop the turnips evenly into small ½-inch dice and to use the broiler on your oven rather than baking them. If you'd like to make this a complete meal, toss some shrimp in the same harissa paste. At the 5-minute mark, move the turnips to one side and add the shrimp, broiling them for 5 minutes.

SERVINGS: 4

DAIRY-FREE
EGG-FREE
NUT-FREE
SOY-FREE
VEGAN

PREP TIME:
10 MINUTES

COOK TIME:
10 MINUTES

TOTAL TIME:
20 MINUTES

COOK TEMPERATURE:
BROIL

MACROS:

Fat: 81%

Carbs: 16%

Protein: 3%

PER SERVING:

Calories: 301

Total Fat: 29 g

Total Carbs: 13 g

Net Carbs: 9 g

Fiber: 4 g

Sugar: 5 g

Sugar Alcohol: 0 g

Protein: 2 g

Cooking spray

2 tablespoons Harissa (page 243)

4 medium turnips, trimmed, peeled, and cut into ½-inch dice (about 4 cups)

1 to 2 tablespoons fresh lemon juice

2 tablespoons chopped fresh parsley

TURN the broiler on high. Spray a large rimmed sheet pan with cooking spray.

In a medium bowl, combine 2 tablespoons of the harissa and the turnips. Mix well to coat.

Arrange the turnips on the prepared pan and broil for 10 minutes, stirring once.

Sprinkle with the lemon juice and parsley and serve.

RAJAS CON CREMA

Not only is this an easy dish, but it's actually gorgeous. The charred peppers, the onion, and the cream sauce just make for a very pretty dish all together. It also keeps well for 3 to 4 days in the refrigerator, making it a great make-ahead dish.

SERVINGS: 4

EGG-FREE
NUT-FREE
SOY-FREE
VEGETARIAN

PREP TIME:
10 MINUTES

COOK TIME:
8 MINUTES

STAND TIME:
5 MINUTES

TOTAL TIME:
23 MINUTES

COOK TEMPERATURE:
BROIL

MACROS:

Fat: 71%

Carbs: 23%

Protein: 6%

PER SERVING:

Calories: 189

Total Fat: 15 g

Total Carbs: 11 g

Net Carbs: 10 g

Fiber: 1 g

Sugar: 1 g

Sugar Alcohol: 0 g

Protein: 3 g

½ red onion, thinly sliced

2 tablespoons vegetable oil

¾ teaspoon kosher salt

4 poblano peppers, cut in half lengthwise and seeded

⅓ cup heavy whipping cream or half-and-half

Juice of ½ lemon

1 tablespoon sour cream

1 teaspoon ground cumin

SET an oven rack 6 inches below the broiler. Preheat the broiler on high.

On a large rimmed sheet pan, toss the onion with 1 tablespoon of the oil and ¼ teaspoon of the salt. Scatter the onions around the pan.

Rub the peppers with the remaining 1 tablespoon oil and sprinkle with ¼ teaspoon of the salt. Arrange the peppers, cut sides down, on the onions. Broil until the tops of the peppers are blistered, about 8 to 10 minutes. Remove from the oven. Cover with foil or a clean cotton kitchen towel; let stand for 5 minutes.

Meanwhile, in a small bowl, stir together the whipping cream, lemon juice, sour cream, cumin, and remaining ¼ teaspoon salt; set aside.

Peel the peppers and slice into long strips. Transfer to a medium bowl and add the onion and cream mixture. Toss to combine.

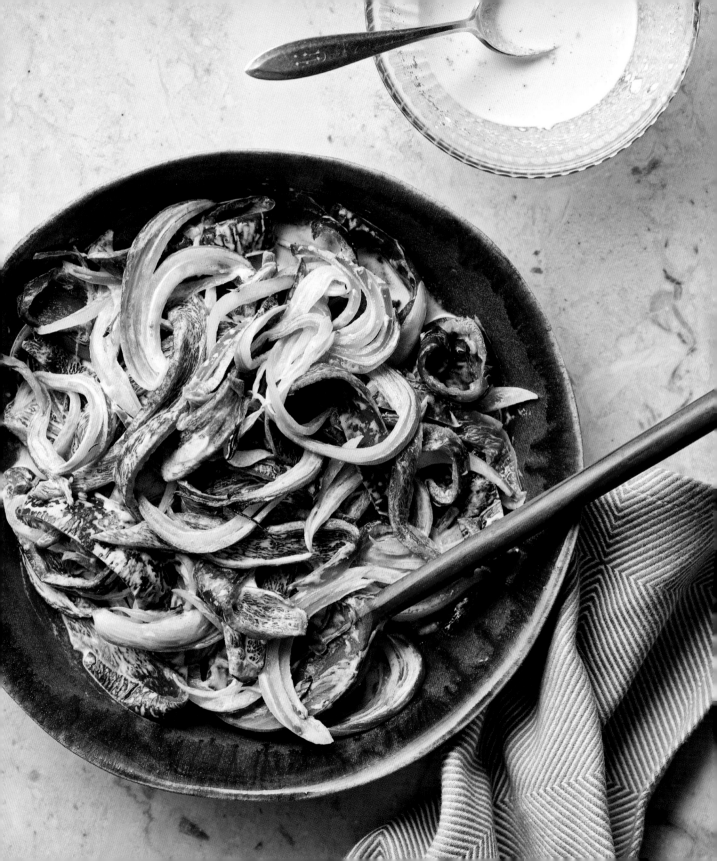

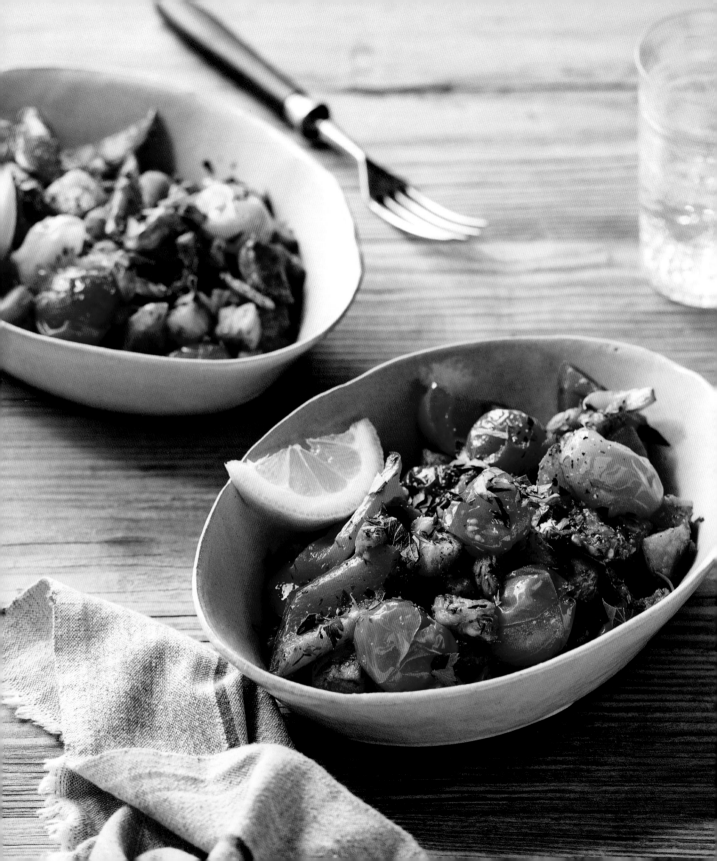

ROASTED RATATOUILLE

Every other roasted eggplant recipe out there tells you it will take a good 30 to 40 minutes to bake and roast. But we aren't going to bake it, we are going to broil it on high heat and be done in 20 minutes. You do need to stir it every 5 minutes to keep it from burning, but the 3 to 4 stirs are well worth it to get dinner on the table quickly.

SERVINGS: 4

DAIRY-FREE
EGG-FREE
NUT-FREE
SOY-FREE
VEGAN

PREP TIME:
10 MINUTES

COOK TIME:
20 MINUTES

TOTAL TIME:
30 MINUTES

COOK TEMPERATURE:
BROIL

MACROS:

Fat: 73%

Carbs: 23%

Protein: 4%

PER SERVING:

Calories: 256

Total Fat: 22 g

Total Carbs: 15 g

Net Carbs: 10 g

Fiber: 5 g

Sugar: 7 g

Sugar Alcohol: 0 g

Protein: 3 g

⅓ cup plus 1 tablespoon extra-virgin olive oil

4 cups peeled and cubed eggplant (¾-inch cubes)

1½ cups chopped bell peppers (red, yellow, or orange)

1½ cups cherry tomatoes

10 cloves garlic, halved lengthwise

2 teaspoons dried oregano

1½ teaspoons kosher salt

1 teaspoon black pepper

1 teaspoon dried thyme

Juice of 1 lemon

¼ cup chopped fresh parsley (optional)

SET the oven rack 6 inches below the broiler. Preheat the broiler on high. Grease a large rimmed sheet pan with the 1 tablespoon olive oil.

In a large bowl, combine the eggplant, bell peppers, tomatoes, garlic, ⅓ cup olive oil, oregano, salt, pepper, and thyme. Toss to combine. Transfer the vegetables to the prepared pan and broil until the vegetables are tender and roasted, about 20 minutes, stirring every 5 minutes to prevent burning.

Sprinkle with lemon juice and parsley, if using.

SHEET PAN OKRA MASALA

If you've never made *bhindi masala* the old-fashioned way, you may not appreciate how easy I have made this. The traditional recipe takes a lot of babysitting, and a ton of oil. This is an easy and fast recipe that still tastes exactly like the traditional recipe. I often eat this hot one day and with yogurt the next day as a cold salad.

SERVINGS: 4

DAIRY-FREE
EGG-FREE
NUT-FREE
SOY-FREE
VEGAN

PREP TIME:
10 MINUTES

COOK TIME:
15 MINUTES

TOTAL TIME:
25 MINUTES

COOK TEMPERATURE:
BROIL

MACROS:

Fat: 50%

Carbs: 41%

Protein: 9%

PER SERVING:

Calories: 120

Total Fat: 7 g

Total Carbs: 14 g

Net Carbs: 9 g

Fiber: 5 g

Sugar: 4 g

Sugar Alcohol: 0 g

Protein: 3 g

1 pound okra (about 4 cups), cut into ¼-inch-thick pieces

1 cup chopped red onion

2 tablespoons vegetable oil or extra-virgin olive oil

1 teaspoon ground turmeric

1 teaspoon kosher salt

1 teaspoon ground cumin

1 teaspoon ground coriander

¼ to ½ teaspoon cayenne

½ cup chopped tomato

1 lemon, quartered

¼ cup chopped fresh cilantro or parsley

PLACE the oven rack two notches below the broiler. Preheat the broiler on high. Line a heavy-duty sheet pan with aluminum foil.

In a large bowl, combine the okra, onion, oil, turmeric, salt, cumin, coriander, and cayenne. Toss to combine.

Arrange the vegetables in a single layer on the prepared sheet. Broil for 15 minutes, stirring once halfway through. With 5 minutes left in the cooking time, clear a space in the middle of the okra mixture and add the tomato. When the tomato has wilted, remove the pan from the oven.

Squeeze the lemon quarters over the vegetables and toss to combine. Sprinkle with the cilantro.

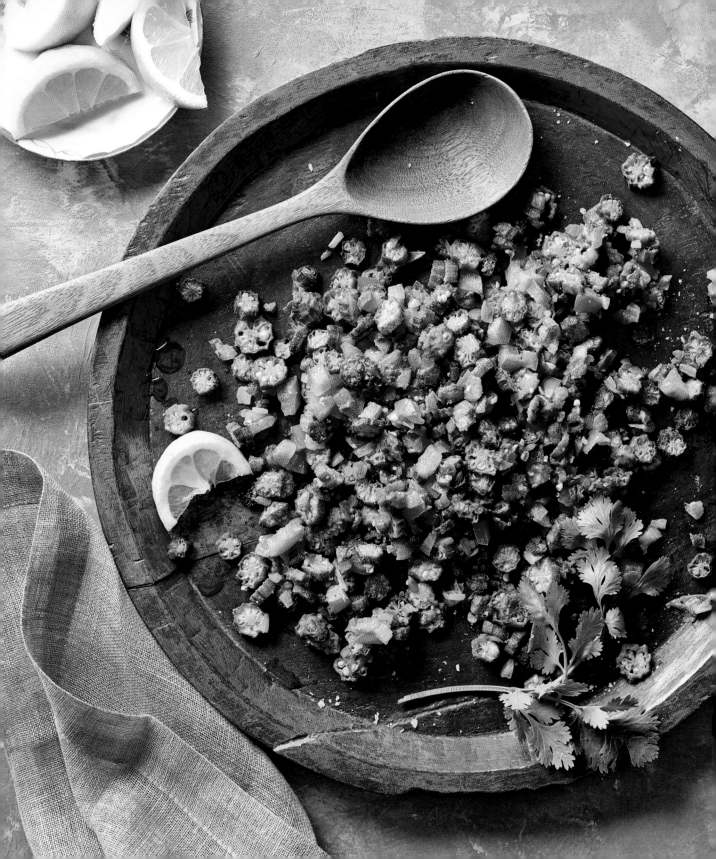

SPICY CREAM OF MUSHROOM SOUP

This tastes like the canned soup you may have grown up with, except with a twist. It's gluten-free and it has just a little kick of spice from one ingredient—the jalapeño! It lends a wonderful flavor to the soup without making it super-spicy.

SERVINGS: 4

EGG-FREE
NUT-FREE
SOY-FREE

PREP TIME:
15 MINUTES

COOK TIME:
15 MINUTES

TOTAL TIME:
30 MINUTES

4 cups sliced button mushrooms

3 cups low-sodium chicken broth or water

2½ cups cauliflower florets

¾ cup diced onion

3 cloves garlic, minced

1 jalapeño, seeded and chopped (optional)

1 teaspoon dried thyme or 3 to 4 sprigs fresh thyme

1 teaspoon kosher salt

1 teaspoon black pepper

1 cup heavy whipping cream

IN A LARGE SAUCEPAN, combine the mushrooms, broth, cauliflower, onion, garlic, jalapeño (if using), thyme, salt, and pepper. Cover and cook over medium heat until the vegetables are cooked through, about 15 minutes.

Using an immersion blender, purée the soup, leaving some mushrooms pieces intact. (If using fresh thyme, remove the sprigs before puréeing.)

Stir in the cream and serve.

NOTES

★ Omit the jalapeño pepper if you want a traditional cream of mushroom soup.

★ This soup tastes FANTASTIC when served chilled as well. Just make ahead of time and serve as a cold soup, which is perfect in summer.

MACROS:

Fat: 72%

Carbs: 18%

Protein: 10%

PER SERVING:

Calories: 262

Total Fat: 22 g

Total Carbs: 13 g

Net Carbs: 10 g

Fiber: 3 g

Sugar: 7 g

Sugar Alcohol: 0 g

Protein: 7 g

VEGETABLES IN CREAM SAUCE

Simple but delicious mixed vegetables, blanketed in a comforting cream sauce? I'm in. This dish goes well with just about any sort of meat you might think of, but you could also add a little queso fresco, paneer cubes, or tofu and call it a full meal.

SERVINGS: 4

NUT-FREE
SOY-FREE

PREP TIME:
10 MINUTES

COOK TIME:
10 MINUTES

TOTAL TIME:
20 MINUTES

MACROS:

Fat: 69%

Carbs: 19%

Protein: 12%

PER SERVING:

Calories: 244

Total Fat: 19 g

Total Carbs: 12 g

Net Carbs: 9 g

Fiber: 3 g

Sugar: 6 g

Sugar Alcohol: 0 g

Protein: 7 g

2 tablespoons butter

1 cup chopped onion (2-inch pieces)

2 cups sliced button mushrooms

1½ cups low-sodium chicken broth

1 cup diced celery

1 cup frozen cut green beans

½ cup diced carrots

1 teaspoon black pepper

1 teaspoon dried thyme

½ teaspoon kosher salt

2 large eggs

½ cup heavy whipping cream

¼ cup chopped fresh parsley

2 tablespoons fresh lemon juice

HEAT a large saucepan over medium-high heat. Add the butter and onion and sauté, stirring frequently, until the onion is translucent, about 3 minutes.

Add the mushrooms, broth, celery, green beans, carrots, pepper, thyme, and salt.

Cover and cook until the vegetables are cooked through, 8 to 10 minutes. Reduce the heat to low.

In a medium bowl, whisk together the eggs, whipping cream, parsley, and lemon juice. Slowly pour this mixture over the vegetables, stirring continuously to prevent the eggs from curdling. Cook over low heat until the sauce has thickened, 1 to 2 minutes. Serve immediately.

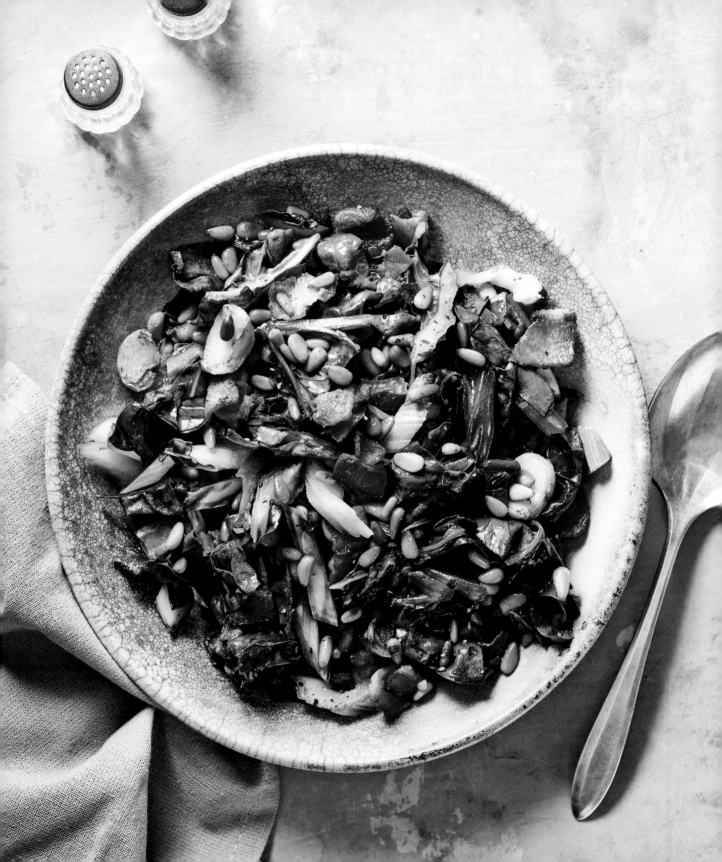

SWISS CHARD WITH GARLIC AND PINE NUTS

Here's what to do with all that lovely Swiss chard you see in the market—or how to make a keto side dish that dresses up any meal in less than 20 minutes. I often just have this for a light supper. You can also add cubed ham or rotisserie chicken to make this a heartier dish.

4 slices bacon, chopped

10 cloves garlic, smashed

¼ cup pine nuts

6 cups chopped Swiss chard

1 teaspoon kosher salt

1 teaspoon black pepper

HEAT a large skillet over medium-high heat. Add the bacon. Cook until the just the edges are crisped, about 5 to 8 minutes.

Add the garlic and press lightly with the back of a spatula. When the garlic is lightly browned, add the pine nuts and mix well. Cook, stirring frequently, until the pine nuts are toasted, 3 to 4 minutes.

Add the chard, ¼ cup water, salt, and pepper. Stir to combine; cover and cook until the chard has just barely wilted, 3 to 4 minutes. (Be careful not to overcook the chard.)

VARIATIONS TO TRY

★ Substitute kale or spinach for the chard and reduce the cook time to 1 to 2 minutes.

★ Substitute walnuts, cashews, or slivered almonds for the pine nuts. Add 1 teaspoon ground cumin

SERVINGS: 4

DAIRY-FREE
EGG-FREE
SOY-FREE

PREP TIME:
5 MINUTES

COOK TIME:
11 MINUTES

TOTAL TIME:
16 MINUTES

MACROS:

Fat: 77%

Carbs: 11%

Protein: 12%

PER SERVING:

Calories: 239

Total Fat: 21 g

Total Carbs: 6 g

Net Carbs: 5 g

Fiber: 1 g

Sugar: 1 g

Sugar Alcohol: 0 g

Protein: 7 g

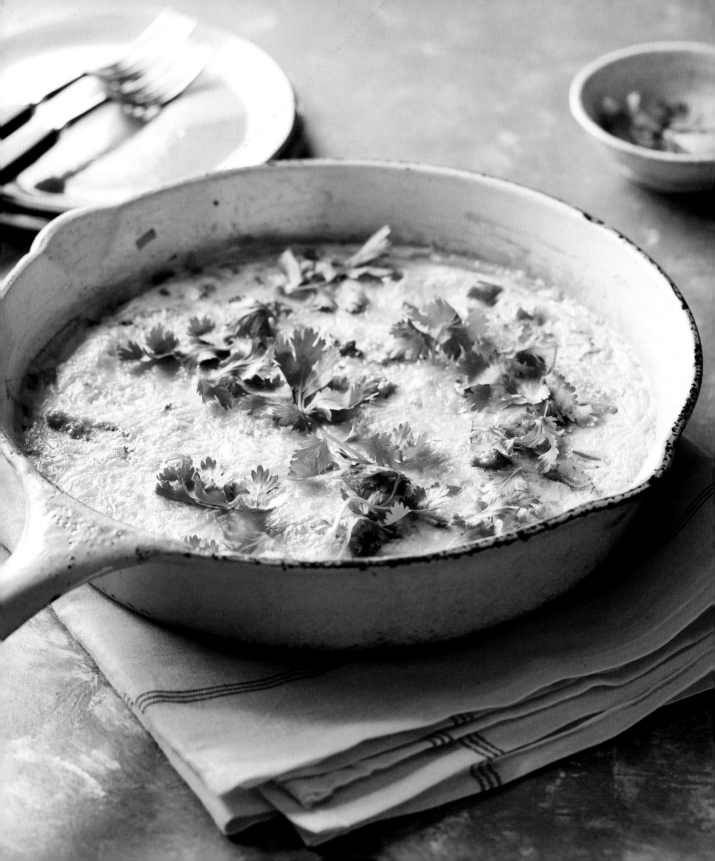

EGGS & CHEESE

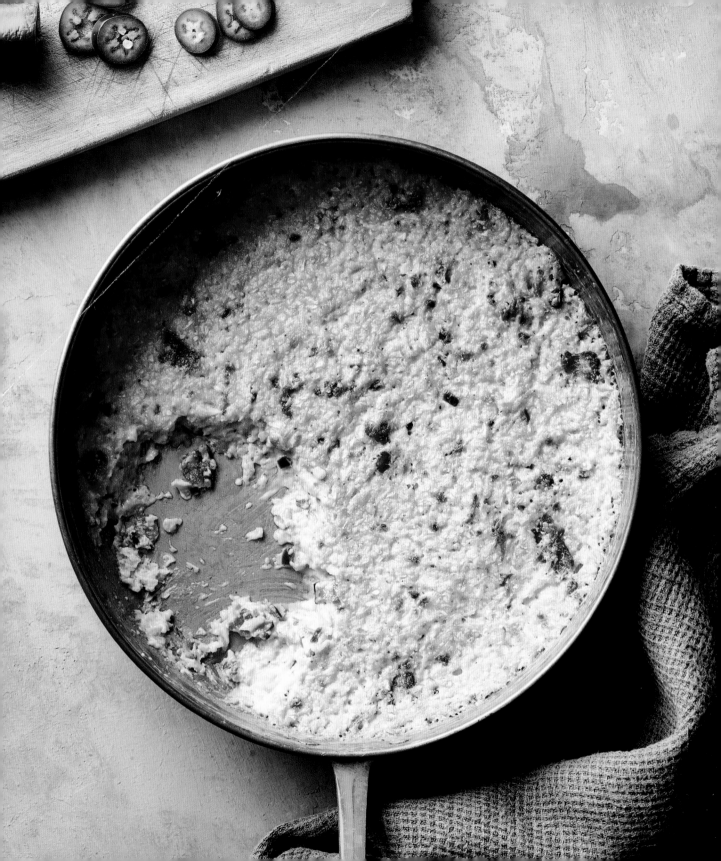

CAULIFLOWER MAC AND CHEESE WITH BACON AND JALAPEÑOS

This is ooey, gooey, creamy, spicy comfort food. I love how easily this goes together. Adjust the number of jalapeños to suit your taste buds. To make it a complete meal, add some chicken tenders after the jalapeños go in. Cook for 5 minutes before adding the cauliflower mixture.

SERVINGS: 6

EGG-FREE
NUT-FREE
SOY-FREE

PREP TIME:
5 MINUTES

COOK TIME:
16 MINUTES

TOTAL TIME:
21 MINUTES

6 slices bacon, chopped

3 cups riced cauliflower

1½ cups Mexican blend cheese or other melting cheese

½ cup heavy whipping cream

4 ounces cream cheese, cubed and softened

1 teaspoon black pepper

½ teaspoon kosher salt

2 jalapeños, seeded and chopped

HEAT a large skillet over high heat. Add the bacon and cook, stirring occasionally, until crisp, 8 to 10 minutes.

Meanwhile, in a large bowl, combine the cauliflower, cheese, whipping cream, cream cheese, pepper, and salt. Mix well.

When the bacon is cooked, add the jalapeños to the pan and cook, stirring, for 1 minute. Add the cauliflower mixture and stir well to combine. Cover and cook over medium-low heat until the cheese has melted, about 8 minutes; stir to combine.

MACROS:

Fat: 81%

Carbs: 5%

Protein: 14%

PER SERVING:

Calories: 408

Total Fat: 37 g

Total Carbs: 6 g

Net Carbs: 5 g

Fiber: 1 g

Sugar: 3 g

Sugar Alcohol: 0 g

Protein: 14 g

NOTE

★ If you'd like, make this in an oven-going skillet and broil for 2 to 3 minutes to lightly brown the top before serving.

⏱ EVEN FASTER TIPS

Use ready-made frozen riced cauliflower. Set it out as you begin to gather ingredients. Don't worry if it isn't fully thawed. You will just have to cook a little longer.

Double the recipe. Cook one batch now and freeze the other uncooked. When ready to cook, thaw and bake as follows: Microwave the bacon; combine the bacon and thawed ingredients in an 8-inch baking dish sprayed with nonstick cooking spray. Bake at 400°F for 15 to 20 minutes.

CHEESE CRISPS

I can't believe I'm giving you a recipe for this, but if you've never made these salty, crispy, crunchy chips, you will thank me. I have these at least 3 to 4 times a week, especially at night when the munchies hit me. Follow this recipe exactly, down to using a paper plate. Do NOT add more cheese, otherwise you won't get a lacy, crispy chip. Melting cheeses work well for this, as do dry cheeses like Parmesan or Asiago.

SERVINGS: 1

EGG-FREE
NUT-FREE
SOY-FREE
VEGETARIAN

PREP TIME:
1 MINUTE

COOK TIME:
90 SECONDS

COOL TIME:
2 MINUTES

TOTAL TIME:
4 MINUTES
30 SECONDS

MACROS:

Fat: 72%

Carbs: 2%

Protein: 26%

PER SERVING:

Calories: 100

Total Fat: 8 g

Total Carbs: 0 g

Net Carbs: 0 g

Fiber: 0 g

Sugar: 0 g

Sugar Alcohol: 0 g

Protein: 7 g

¼ cup shredded Mexican blend cheese or Parmesan cheese

SPREAD THE CHEESE on an 8-inch paper plate. Microwave on high until the cheese is melted and browned, about 90 seconds.

Gently lift up the edge to separate the cheese from the plate. Allow the cheese to cool completely to crisp up.

Troubleshooting: If your chip isn't crispy but instead turns out thick and bendy, you've used too much cheese in one go. Make two plates if you need to, but don't overcrowd one plate.

If your chip isn't well-browned, it won't be as crisp. If you rush it and don't let it cool, it won't be as crisp. It's only three minutes, so be patient and do it right. You can thank me later.

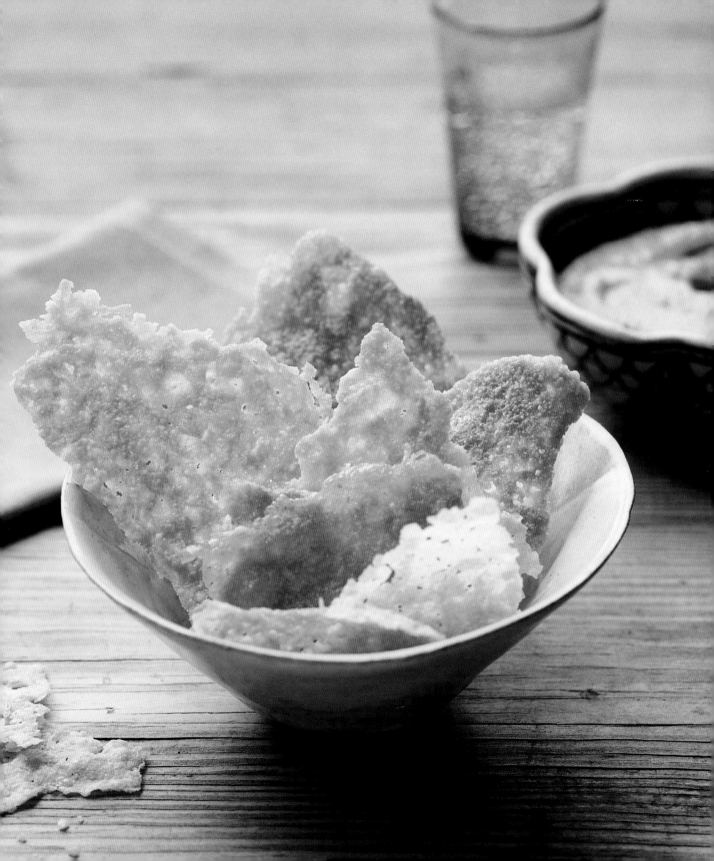

HOT AND SOUR EGG DROP SOUP

This soup combines two classic Chinese food recipes into one. If you do not have Chinese rice vinegar, use regular white vinegar but add a little Swerve for the sweeter taste that rice vinegar has. If you need to increase the protein or make it more of a meal, you can add diced chicken, tofu, or thinly sliced pork to the broth as it boils. Allow the meats to cook before you add the eggs.

SERVINGS: 4

DAIRY-FREE
NUT-FREE

PREP TIME:
10 MINUTES

COOK TIME:
5 MINUTES

STAND TIME:
2 MINUTES

TOTAL TIME:
17 MINUTES

MACROS:

Fat: 52%

Carbs: 11%

Protein: 37%

PER SERVING:

Calories: 83

Total Fat: 5 g

Total Carbs: 2 g

Net Carbs: 2 g

Fiber: 0 g

Sugar: 1 g

Sugar Alcohol: 0 g

Protein: 8 g

4 cups low-sodium chicken broth

4½ teaspoons Chinese rice vinegar

1 tablespoon soy sauce

1 tablespoon Chinese black vinegar

1 tablespoon chili oil (optional)

¼ teaspoon kosher salt

½ teaspoon xanthan gum

4 large eggs, lightly beaten

HEAT a large saucepan over medium heat. Combine the broth, rice vinegar, soy sauce, black vinegar, chili oil (if using), salt, and xanthan gum. Bring to a boil and cook for 1 to 2 minutes.

Slowly pour in the beaten eggs; stir around the pot three times. Turn off the flame; cover. Allow to stand 2 minutes before serving.

VARIATION TO TRY

★ If you can't find Chinese black vinegar, balsamic vinegar works surprisingly well.

EVEN FASTER TIP

Make a double batch. Doctor it up the second day with cooked rotisserie chicken and some green onions.

BROCCOLI CHEESE SOUP

If you follow my advice and keep frozen broccoli florets in the freezer, this soup will come together in no time at all. Use low-sodium broth if you can find it, or just water if you can't—otherwise you may end up with a soup that is too salty. If using water, add salt to taste.

1 tablespoon butter

½ cup diced onion

4 cloves garlic, sliced

4 cups broccoli florets, frozen or fresh

3 cups low-sodium chicken broth or vegetable broth

1 teaspoon black pepper

2 ounces cream cheese, diced

½ cup heavy whipping cream

2 cups shredded cheddar cheese

2 to 3 dashes hot sauce (optional)

HEAT a large saucepan over medium heat; add the butter. Add the onion and garlic. Cook and stir for 30 seconds.

Add the broccoli, broth, and pepper. Bring to a simmer and cook until the broccoli is tender, 8 to 10 minutes. Turn the heat to low. Use an immersion blender to purée the soup, leaving some of florets whole. (Or just mash using the back of a spoon.)

Turn the heat to medium; add the cream cheese and stir to melt. Bring mixture to a boil, then turn the heat to low and add the cream. Add the cheddar cheese, one handful at a time, and stir until each handful is melted.

Add hot sauce, if desired, and serve.

EVEN FASTER TIP

Use frozen, precut onion in addition to the frozen broccoli to make this go even faster.

SERVINGS: 6

EGG-FREE
NUT-FREE
SOY-FREE

PREP TIME:
10 MINUTES

COOK TIME:
15 MINUTES

TOTAL TIME:
25 MINUTES

MACROS:

Fat: 73%

Carbs: 11%

Protein: 16%

PER SERVING:

Calories: 303

Total Fat: 25 g

Total Carbs: 9 g

Net Carbs: 7 g

Fiber: 2 g

Sugar: 3 g

Sugar Alcohol: 0 g

Protein: 12 g

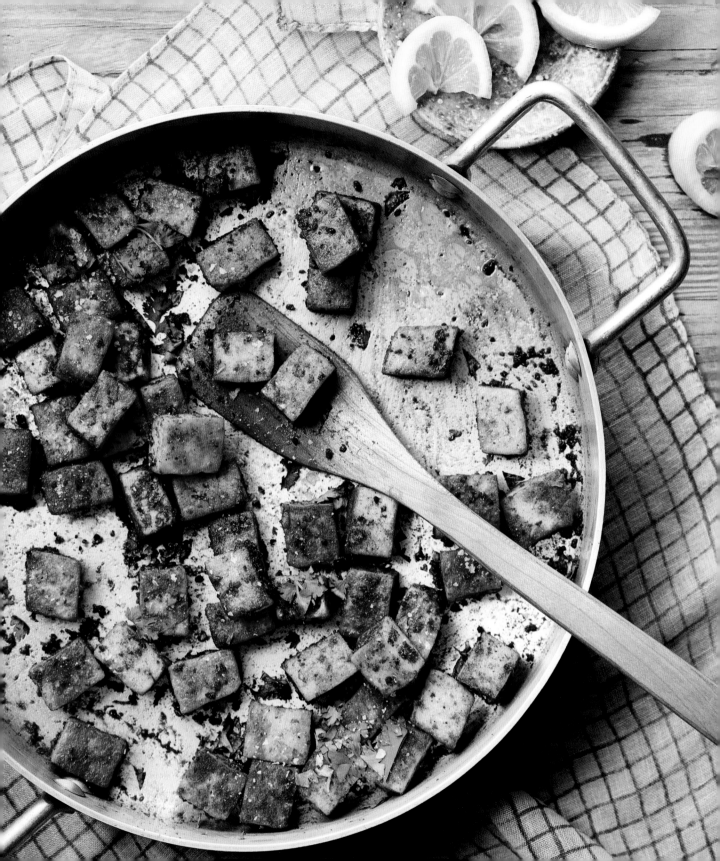

PANEER TIKKA

Paneer is a great quick-made Indian cheese that can be found in Indian grocery stores. You can also find a recipe for homemade paneer on my blog twosleevers.com and I would highly recommend you try that one. But if you can't find it near you, a Mexican queso fresco is quite similar. You just want a cheese that will soften, but not melt into a puddle basically and you will be all set. This paneer is best eaten the day it's made. You can however, marinate it for up to 2 to 3 days in the fridge and only remove and cook as much as you need that day.

SERVINGS: 4

EGG-FREE
NUT-FREE
SOY-FREE
VEGETARIAN

PREP TIME:
5 MINUTES

COOK TIME:
4 MINUTES

TOTAL TIME:
9 MINUTES

MACROS:

Fat: 72%

Carbs: 7%

Protein: 21%

PER SERVING:

Calories: 335

Total Fat: 28 g

Total Carbs: 6 g

Net Carbs: 5 g

Fiber: 1 g

Sugar: 3 g

Sugar Alcohol: 0 g

Protein: 18 g

3 cups cubed paneer

¼ cup chopped fresh cilantro

1 tablespoon vegetable oil

3 cloves garlic, minced

1 tablespoon minced fresh ginger

2 teaspoons Indian Garam Masala (page 244)

1 teaspoon ground turmeric

1 teaspoon ground cumin

1 teaspoon ground coriander

1 teaspoon smoked paprika

1 teaspoon kosher salt

½ teaspoon cayenne pepper

1 tablespoon ghee or Homemade Ghee (page 239)

1 lemon, halved

IN A LARGE BOWL, gently combine the paneer, cilantro, vegetable oil, garlic, ginger, garam masala, turmeric, cumin, coriander, paprika, salt, and cayenne pepper. Be sure to not break the paneer.

Heat a large skillet over high heat; add the ghee. Once the ghee is melted, add the paneer cubes in a single layer. Sear for 3 to 4 minutes, turning once halfway through cooking time. Once both sides are seared, remove from the heat.

Squeeze the lemon halves over the paneer.

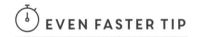 EVEN FASTER TIP

Double the recipe and place half into a plastic zipper bag after step 1. Marinate for up to 2 to 3 days. Remove when ready to cook.

SOUTHWESTERN FRITTATA

This is a great basic frittata recipe that you can mix up and make in a variety of ways. As long as you precook the vegetables to get rid of all the excess moisture, you will get a great texture. Precooking the eggs in the skillet a little will help to cook the eggs faster, rather than putting the uncooked eggs in the oven. This makes a dense, fillings-packed egg dish. If you'd like it eggier, add 2 more eggs for a more custardy version. You could also make this into frittata muffins.

SERVINGS: 6

NUT-FREE
SOY-FREE

PREP TIME:
10 MINUTES

COOK TIME:
12 MINUTES

TOTAL TIME:
22 MINUTES

COOK TEMPERATURE:
BROIL

MACROS:

Fat: 67%

Carbs: 6%

Protein: 27%

PER SERVING:

Calories: 311

Total Fat: 23 g

Total Carbs: 5 g

Net Carbs: 4 g

Fiber: 1 g

Sugar: 3 g

Sugar Alcohol: 0 g

Protein: 21 g

½ pound bulk breakfast sausage

8 large eggs

½ cup half-and-half

½ teaspoon kosher salt

1 cup chopped bell pepper

½ cup chopped onion

¼ cup chopped fresh cilantro or parsley, plus more for serving

1 jalapeño, seeded and diced, or 1 (4.5-ounce) can mild green chiles, drained

1 teaspoon ground cumin

1 cup shredded Mexican cheese or pepper jack cheese

SET THE OVEN RACK 6 inches below the broiler. Preheat the broiler on high.

Heat a large ovenproof skillet over medium-high heat. Add the sausage and cook, breaking it up with a wooden spoon and stirring, until it is about halfway cooked, 4 to 5 minutes.

Meanwhile, in a large bowl, beat the eggs, half-and-half, and salt together. Set aside.

Add the bell pepper, onion, the ¼ cup chopped cilantro, jalapeño, and cumin to the sausage. Cook, stirring, until the vegetables have wilted and the sausage is cooked through, 3 to 4 minutes.

Turn the heat to medium-low. Pour the egg mixture into the skillet and stir a few times, until the eggs have cooked a little.

Shake the pan to redistribute the eggs evenly. Sprinkle the cheese on the eggs. Place the skillet under the broiler until the cheese has melted and the eggs have cooked through, 3 to 4 minutes.

Remove the pan from the oven. Cover and allow the eggs to finish cooking for 2 to 3 minutes. Sprinkle with additional cilantro. Cut into wedges and serve.

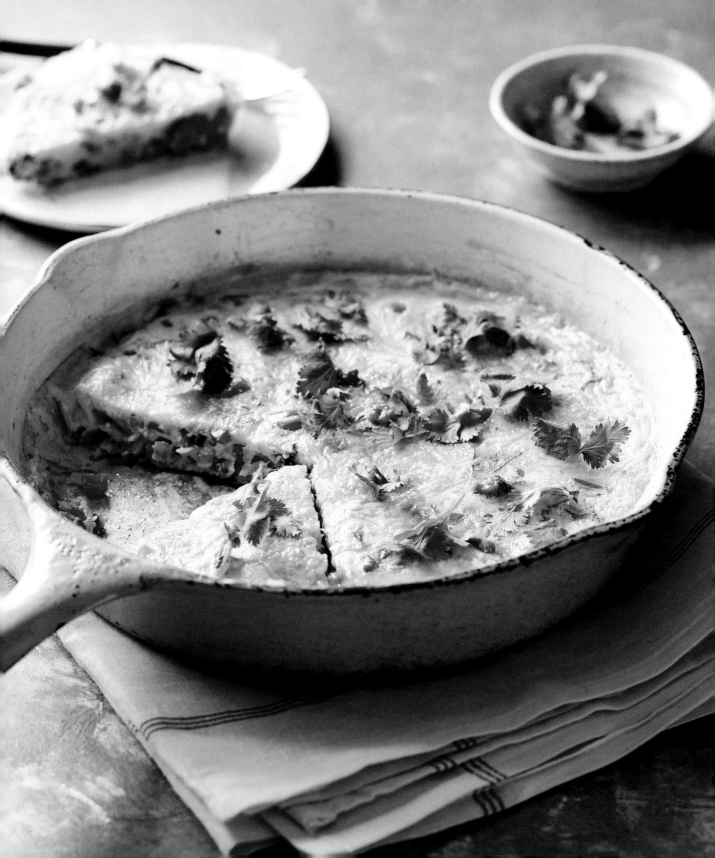

QUESO FUNDIDO

See this recipe right here? This one alone is a great reason to love a keto way of eating. Cheese, sausage, and cream together, eaten with crunchy vegetables is such an easy supper and feels utterly decadent. Be sure to use Mexican-style chorizo—which is a crumbly sausage—not the dried Spanish variety. If you can't get it where you live, any type of fresh sausage will do.

SERVINGS: 6

EGG-FREE
NUT-FREE
SOY-FREE

PREP TIME:
5 MINUTES

COOK TIME:
20 MINUTES

STAND TIME:
1 MINUTE

TOTAL TIME:
26 MINUTES

MACROS:

Fat: 71%

Carbs: 8%

Protein: 21%

PER SERVING:

Calories: 465

Total Fat: 38 g

Total Carbs: 10 g

Net Carbs: 8 g

Fiber: 2 g

Sugar: 3 g

Sugar Alcohol: 0 g

Protein: 25 g

8 ounces Mexican-style chorizo, casings removed

½ cup chopped onion

6 cloves garlic, minced

3 jalapeños, seeded and chopped

½ cup chopped tomato

3 teaspoons ground cumin

¾ cup heavy whipping cream

3 cups grated Oaxaca cheese or mozzarella

¼ cup chopped fresh cilantro or parsley

1 large bell pepper, stemmed, seeded, and thickly sliced, for serving

8 stalks celery, cut into 3-inch pieces, for serving

HEAT a large saucepan over medium heat. Add the chorizo, onion, garlic, and jalapeños and cook, stirring, until chorizo is browned and cooked through, about 8 minutes. Add the tomato and cumin and cook, stirring, for 2 to 3 minutes. Stir in the cream.

Slowly add the cheese, a handful at a time, stirring continuously to keep it from seizing. When the cheese has almost completely melted, remove the pan from the heat. Cover and let rest for 1 minute to finish melting.

Sprinkle with the cilantro and serve with sliced bell peppers and/or celery for dipping.

EASY KETO EGG RECIPES

Get into the habit of making one large roast chicken and a dozen boiled eggs over the weekend, and you will never lack for snacks, quick meals, and portable lunches. These simple but tasty recipes are perfect for those nights when you stand in front of your fridge, exhausted, hungry, and are tempted to dial for takeout. You can make any of these faster than you could order a pizza! You have no excuse now.

My favorite way to make hard-cooked eggs is in an air fryer. Use 250°F for 18 minutes, followed by an ice bath (for the eggs, not for you), and you end up with perfectly cooked eggs—and no pots to wash!

My favorite way to eat boiled eggs has become very popular in my Facebook group: chopped hard boiled eggs, melted butter, salt, and pepper. SO good! Sounds like nothing, tastes like crazy good comfort food. I hope you try that one for sure!

(Chart begins on page 114.)

NAME	EGGS/OTHER PROTEINS	FAT	SEASONINGS/CONDIMENTS
QUICK EGG SALAD	2 hard-cooked eggs, peeled and chopped	2 Tbsp mayonnaise	½ tsp whole-grain mustard ¼ fresh lemon juice Pinch each salt and pepper
BUFFALO DEVILED EGGS	2 hard-cooked eggs, peeled and halved	1 Tbsp mayonnaise 1 Tbsp crumbled blue cheese	½ tsp fresh lemon juice ½ tsp yellow mustard Pinch each salt and pepper
GUACAMOLE DEVILED EGGS	2 hard-cooked eggs, peeled and halved	1 Tbsp mayonnaise 1 Tbsp guacamole	½ tsp fresh lemon juice Pinch each salt and pepper
EGG AND AVOCADO BOWL	2 hard-cooked eggs, peeled and chopped	½ ripe avocado, coarsely chopped	1 Tbsp vinaigrette Pinch each salt and pepper
EGG AND AVOCADO WRAPS	1 hard-cooked egg, peeled and sliced	2 Tbsp guacamole	Pinch each salt and pepper
EGG AND RADISH WRAPS	1 hard-cooked egg, peeled and sliced	1 Tbsp mayonnaise	Pinch of coarse salt
HARD-COOKED EGG WITH MUSTARD AND HERBS	2 hard-cooked eggs, peeled and halved		Whole-grain mustard Pinch each salt and pepper
BUTTERED HARD-COOKED EGGS	2 hard-cooked eggs, peeled and diced	1 Tbsp melted butter	Pinch each salt and pepper
GREEN SALAD WITH CRUMBLED EGGS AND BACON	2 hard-cooked eggs, peeled and grated on a box grater 1 piece cooked and crumbled bacon		Vinaigrette Pinch each salt and pepper
SALMON SALAD BOATS WITH CURRIED EGGS	1 (2.5-ounce) package salmon 1 hard-cooked egg, peeled and sliced	1 Tbsp mayonnaise	Pinch of salt Curry powder

VEGETABLES/HERBS	METHOD
2 Tbsp finely minced celery 1 green onion, sliced 1 lettuce leaf	Stir together everything except the lettuce leaf. Scoop into lettuce.
1 Tbsp finely diced celery	Mash the egg yolks with the remaining ingredients. Spoon evenly into egg whites.
	Mash the egg yolks with the mayonnaise, guacamole, lemon juice, and salt and pepper. Spoon evenly into egg whites.
2 cherry tomatoes, quartered 1 green onion, trimmed and sliced 1 heaping Tbsp finely chopped red bell pepper	Toss everything together.
2 butter lettuce leaves	Spread the guacamole on the lettuce leaves. Top with egg slices. Sprinkle with salt and pepper.
2 butter lettuce leaves 2 radishes, trimmed and sliced	Spread lettuce leaves with mayonnaise. Top with egg and radish slices. Sprinkle with salt.
Chopped fresh herbs, such as parsley, chives, or basil	Spread egg halves with mustard. Sprinkle with salt and pepper. Top with fresh herbs.
	Drizzle eggs with melted butter. Sprinkle with salt and pepper.
Salad greens or baby spinach	Lightly dress the greens with vinaigrette. Top with crumbled egg and bacon. Sprinkle with salt and pepper.
2 quarters of a red, yellow, or orange bell pepper	Stir together the salmon, mayonnaise, and a pinch each of salt and pepper. Scoop onto the pepper quarters. Top with sliced egg. Sprinkle with salt and curry powder.

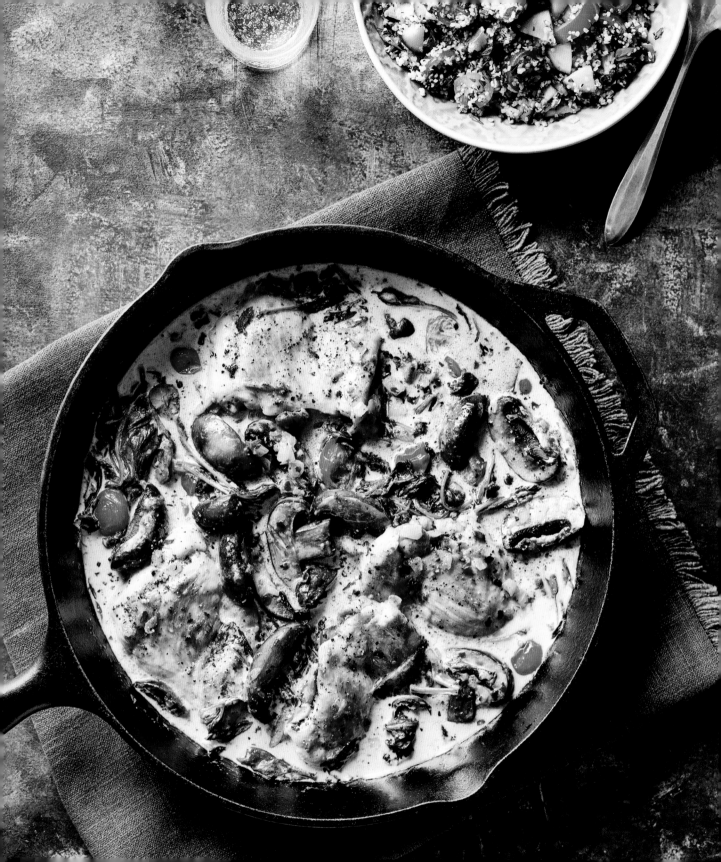

CHICKEN

ARTICHOKE CHICKEN SOUP

Artichokes, spinach, and cheese don't just belong in a dip. Add some chicken for a heartier meal and enjoy this soup instead. Like many soups, this gets better as it sits, so make extra and take it for lunch the next day.

1 pound chicken tenders, cut into bite-size pieces

1 (12-ounce) package frozen chopped spinach

1 (8-ounce) jar marinated artichokes, undrained

3 cups low-sodium chicken broth

½ cup chopped onion

3 cloves garlic, minced

1 teaspoon Italian seasoning

½ teaspoon red pepper flakes

1 teaspoon kosher salt

½ teaspoon black pepper

1 tablespoon fresh lemon juice

½ cup shredded Parmesan cheese

IN A LARGE SAUCEPAN, combine the chicken, spinach, artichokes, broth, onion, garlic, Italian seasoning, red pepper flakes, salt, and pepper. Bring to a boil over high heat. Reduce heat and simmer for 20 minutes. Stir in the lemon juice and Parmesan cheese.

SERVINGS: 4

EGG-FREE
NUT-FREE
SOY-FREE

PREP TIME:
5 MINUTES

COOK TIME:
20 MINUTES

TOTAL TIME:
25 MINUTES

MACROS:

Fat: 30%

Carbs: 17%

Protein: 53%

PER SERVING:

Calories: 274

Total Fat: 9 g

Total Carbs: 11 g

Net Carbs: 8 g

Fiber: 3 g

Sugar: 1 g

Sugar Alcohol: 0 g

Protein: 34 g

BUFFALO CHICKEN CASSEROLE

Creamy and spicy things are such a great food sensation, and this is yet another quickly put together dish. I'm told this also microwaves very well—you could mix everything up and cover it and put it in the fridge. When it's time to eat, remove your portion and zap it. Or cook as directed so you will have plenty to share with others.

Cooking spray

4 cups shredded rotisserie chicken

½ cup chopped onion

¼ cup heavy whipping cream

¼ cup hot wing sauce

¼ cup crumbled blue cheese

2 ounces cream cheese, diced

¼ teaspoon kosher salt

⅛ teaspoon black pepper

¼ cup chopped green onions, white and green parts, for garnish

Celery sticks, for serving (optional)

PREHEAT oven to 400°F. Spray an 8 × 8-inch baking dish with cooking spray.

In the prepared dish, stir together the chicken, onion, cream, wing sauce, blue cheese, cream cheese, salt, and pepper.

Bake for 15 minutes or until heated through and bubbling. Remove from the oven and stir well to mix cheeses. Cover with foil and allow to rest for 2 to 3 minutes.

Garnish with the chopped green onions and serve with celery sticks, if desired.

SERVINGS: 4 AS A MAIN COURSE, OR 8 AS AN APPETIZER

EGG-FREE
NUT-FREE
SOY-FREE

PREP TIME:
10 MINUTES

COOK TIME:
15 MINUTES

STAND TIME:
2 MINUTES

TOTAL TIME:
27 MINUTES

COOK TEMPERATURE:
400°F

MACROS:

Fat: 52%

Carbs: 3%

Protein: 45%

PER SERVING:

Calories: 424

Total Fat: 25 g

Total Carbs: 4 g

Net Carbs: 3 g

Fiber: 1 g

Sugar: 2 g

Sugar Alcohol: 0 g

Protein: 48 g

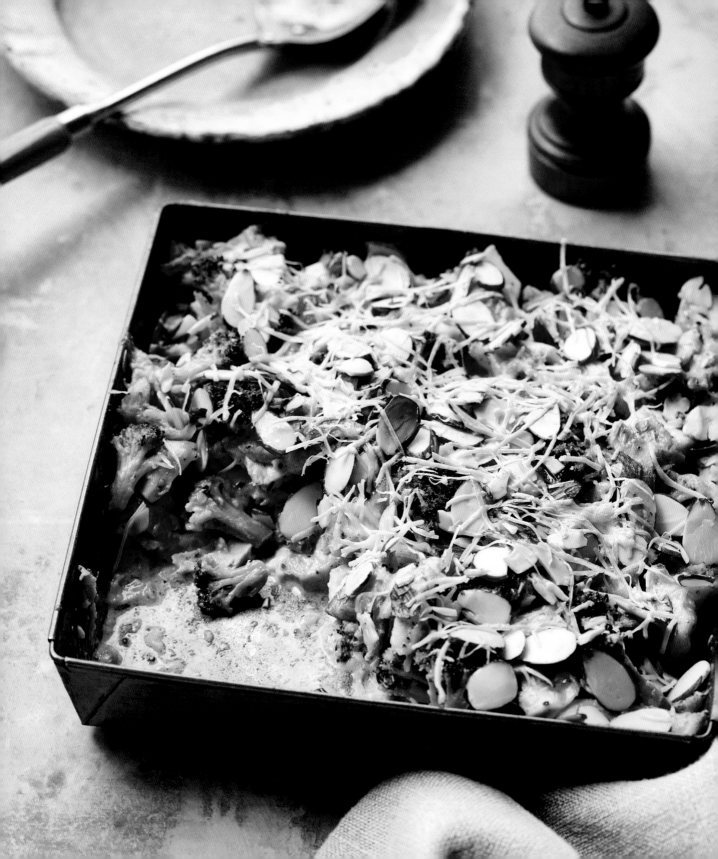

BROCCOLI CHICKEN BAKE

If you're looking for dishes for using leftover rotisserie chicken, this is an easy one. With the toasted almonds on top, not only is it a quick and tasty dish, it's also actually pretty enough to serve for company.

Cooking spray

4 cups frozen broccoli florets, thawed

3 cups chopped rotisserie chicken

1½ cups shredded cheddar cheese

½ cup heavy whipping cream

2 teaspoons chicken bouillon paste (optional)

1 teaspoon black pepper

½ cup sliced almonds

¼ cup shredded Parmesan cheese

PREHEAT the oven to 400°F. Spray a 9-inch square baking dish or 9-inch pie plate with cooking spray.

In a large bowl, stir together the broccoli, chicken, cheese, cream, bouillon paste (if using), and pepper.

Pour the mixture into the prepared pan. Top with the almonds and Parmesan cheese.

Bake until hot and bubbling, 15 to 20 minutes.

Let stand 5 minutes before serving.

SERVINGS: 4

EGG-FREE
SOY-FREE

PREP TIME:
5 MINUTES

COOK TIME:
15 MINUTES

STAND TIME:
5 MINUTES

TOTAL TIME:
25 MINUTES

COOK TEMPERATURE:
400°F

MACROS:

Fat: 61%

Carbs: 6%

Protein: 33%

PER SERVING:

Calories: 608

Total Fat: 41 g

Total Carbs: 9 g

Net Carbs: 5 g

Fiber: 4 g

Sugar: 4 g

Sugar Alcohol: 0 g

Protein: 50 g

CHICKEN BIRYANI

For my last meal on this earth, I want Chicken Biryani. That's how much I love biryanis. But of course, the rice is an absolute nonstarter for me. This low-carb version definitely tastes like the real thing—except no carbs and you're also not dirtying every pot in the house.

SERVINGS: 4

DAIRY-FREE
EGG-FREE
NUT-FREE
SOY-FREE

PREP TIME:
10 MINUTES

COOK TIME:
20 MINUTES

TOTAL TIME:
30 MINUTES

MACROS:

Fat: 50%

Carbs: 11%

Protein: 39%

PER SERVING:

Calories: 214

Total Fat: 12 g

Total Carbs: 6 g

Net Carbs: 4 g

Fiber: 2 g

Sugar: 2 g

Sugar Alcohol: 0 g

Protein: 21 g

FOR THE CHICKEN

1 teaspoon Homemade Ghee (page 239) or ghee

1 pound ground chicken

1 teaspoon kosher salt

1 teaspoon Indian Garam Masala (page 244)

½ teaspoon ground turmeric

½ teaspoon ground coriander

¼ teaspoon ground cumin

FOR THE VEGETABLES

1 teaspoon Homemade Ghee (page 239) or ghee

1 small red onion, thinly sliced

1 jalapeño, seeded and chopped

1 teaspoon ginger-garlic paste (or ½ teaspoon minced garlic + ½ teaspoon minced ginger)

½ cup chopped fresh cilantro

¼ cup chopped fresh mint

2 cups riced cauliflower

Kosher salt

FOR THE CHICKEN: Heat a large deep skillet over medium-high heat; add the ghee. Once the ghee is melted, add the chicken and cook, breaking it up with a wooden spoon, until chicken is cooked through, about 5 minutes.

Add the salt, garam masala, turmeric, coriander, and cumin and stir to combine. Cook, stirring frequently, until the liquid evaporates, about 3 minutes. Transfer the chicken to a bowl; set aside.

FOR THE VEGETABLES: Heat a large skillet over medium-high heat; add the ghee. Once the ghee is melted, add the onion and cook, stirring, until the onion is brown at the edges, about 5 minutes.

Add the jalapeño and the ginger-garlic paste and cook for 1 to 2 minutes. Add ½ cup water and stir to deglaze the pan, scraping up the brown bits from the bottom.

Add the cooked chicken, cilantro, mint, and riced cauliflower. Mix well and cover. Turn the heat to low and simmer, allowing the flavors to blend and the cauliflower to cook until crisp-tender, 5 minutes. (Be sure to not let the cauliflower become mushy.)

Season with salt to taste.

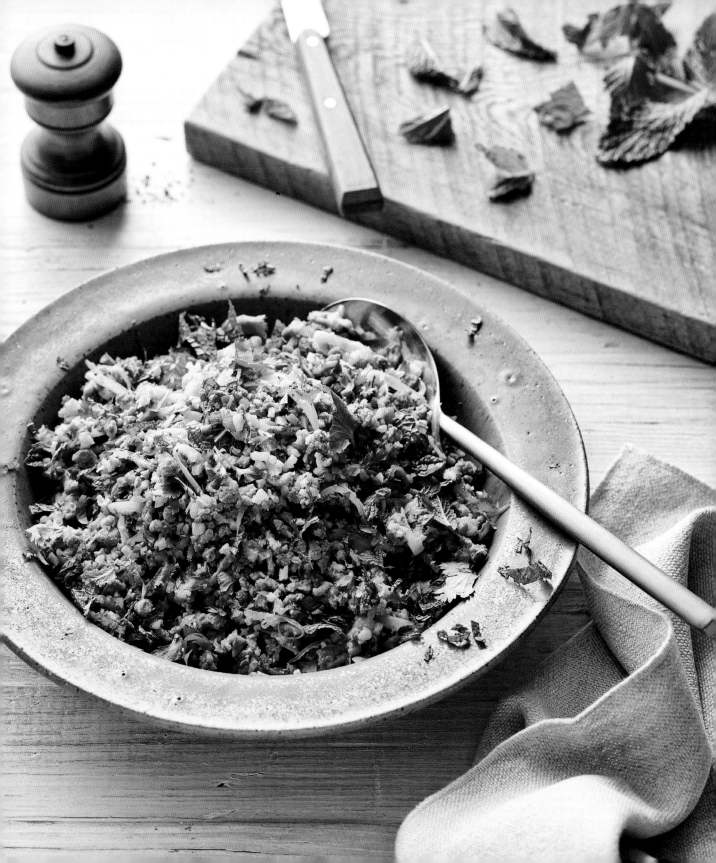

CHICKEN CORDON BLEU CASSEROLE

This is a great way to use up leftover rotisserie chicken. Add a little deli ham and some staples from the fridge and pantry, and no one will know how easy it was to put this tasty delight together. The nutmeg really makes this dish shine, so don't overlook that.

SERVINGS: 6

EGG-FREE
NUT-FREE
SOY-FREE

PREP TIME:
10 MINUTES

COOK TIME:
20 MINUTES

TOTAL TIME:
30 MINUTES

COOK TEMPERATURE:
400°F

MACROS:

Fat: 50%

Carbs: 5%

Protein: 45%

PER SERVING:

Calories: 318

Total Fat: 17 g

Total Carbs: 4 g

Net Carbs: 4 g

Fiber: 0 g

Sugar: 3 g

Sugar Alcohol: 0 g

Protein: 34 g

Cooking spray

3 cups diced cooked chicken

1½ cups diced ham

¾ cup half-and-half

1 teaspoon black pepper

½ teaspoon ground nutmeg

8 slices Swiss cheese

PREHEAT the oven to 400°F. Spray an 8 × 8-inch square baking pan with cooking spray.

In a large bowl, toss together the chicken, ham, half-and-half, pepper, and nutmeg.

Place half of the chicken mixture in the pan. Tear up 3 slices of the cheese and scatter over the top of the chicken mixture. Top with the remaining chicken mixture. Layer the remaining slices of Swiss cheese on top.

Bake for 20 minutes or until heated through and bubbling; serve hot.

EVEN FASTER TIP

This recipe freezes well and tastes even better the next day.

CHICKEN POT PIE SOUP

Not only is this a fantastic substitute for chicken pot pie but this soup also freezes very well.

SERVINGS: 4

EGG-FREE
NUT-FREE
SOY-FREE

PREP TIME:
10 MINUTES

COOK TIME:
20 MINUTES

TOTAL TIME:
30 MINUTES

MACROS:

Fat: 64%

Carbs: 7%

Protein: 29%

PER SERVING:

Calories: 507

Total Fat: 36 g

Total Carbs: 9 g

Net Carbs: 7 g

Fiber: 2 g

Sugar: 4 g

Sugar Alcohol: 0 g

Protein: 37 g

2 tablespoons butter

1 cup diced celery

½ cup chopped onion

3 cloves garlic, minced

3 cups diced rotisserie chicken

3 cups low-sodium chicken broth

1 cup frozen cut green beans

½ cup sliced carrots

⅓ cup frozen green peas (optional)

1 teaspoon black pepper

1 teaspoon dried thyme

¼ to ½ teaspoon kosher salt

1 cup heavy whipping cream

¼ teaspoon xanthan gum

HEAT a large saucepan over medium heat; add the butter. Once the butter has melted, add the celery, onion, and garlic and cook, stirring, until the onion is translucent, about 2 minutes.

Add the chicken, broth, green beans, carrots, peas (if using), pepper, thyme, and salt. Bring to a boil. Reduce heat to a simmer and cook, stirring occasionally, until the vegetables are done, about 10 minutes.

Pour in the cream in a slow and steady stream. Stir in the xanthan gum. Bring the soup to a boil. Reduce heat and simmer for 5 minutes.

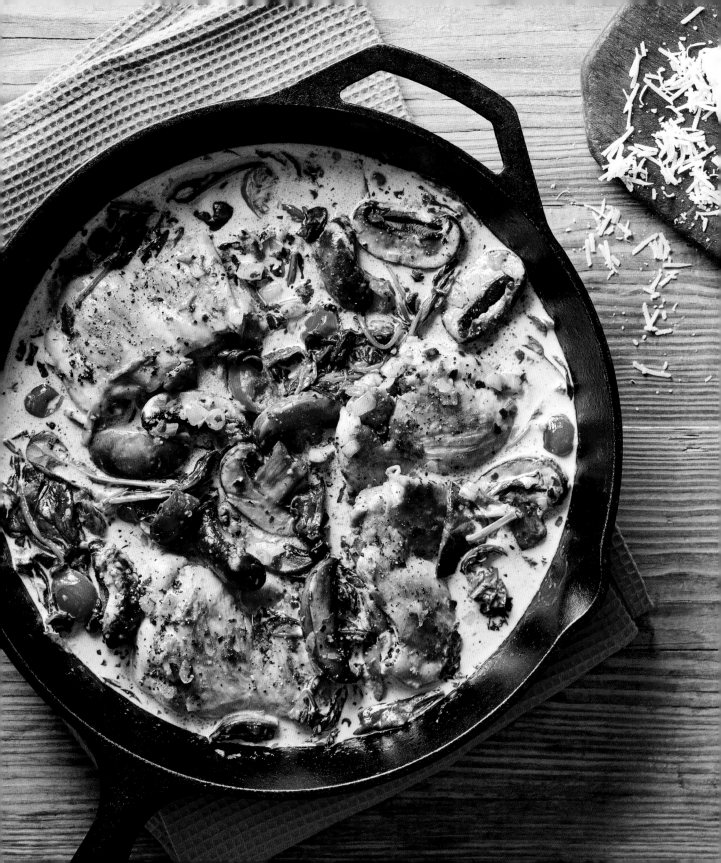

CREAMY TUSCAN CHICKEN

My friend John, who tests recipes for me, wrote "HOME RUN" on this recipe! "AMAZING FLAVOR," he said! And I trust John, who has been cooking for 40+ years. So, let's trust him with this one—make it immediately!

SERVINGS: 4

EGG-FREE
NUT-FREE
SOY-FREE

PREP TIME:
10 MINUTES

COOK TIME:
20 MINUTES

TOTAL TIME:
30 MINUTES

MACROS:

Fat: 67%

Carbs: 8%

Protein: 25%

PER SERVING:

Calories: 486

Total Fat: 36 g

Total Carbs: 10 g

Net Carbs: 8 g

Fiber: 2 g

Sugar: 4 g

Sugar Alcohol: 0 g

Protein: 31 g

2 tablespoons butter

½ cup chopped onion

3 cloves garlic, minced

1 teaspoon red pepper flakes (optional)

1 pound boneless, skinless chicken thighs

4 cups baby spinach

1 cup sliced mushrooms

1 cup cherry tomatoes, halved

1 teaspoon Italian seasoning

1 teaspoon black pepper

½ teaspoon kosher salt

1 cup heavy whipping cream

¾ cup grated Parmesan cheese

HEAT a large skillet over medium-low heat; add the butter. Once the butter is melted, add the onion, garlic, and red pepper flakes, if using. Cook, stirring, until the onions are coated, about 30 seconds.

Add the chicken, spinach, mushrooms, tomatoes, Italian seasoning, pepper, and salt. Mix well.

Pour in the cream and stir to combine. Cover and cook until the chicken has reached an internal temperature of 165°F, about 15 minutes.

Stir in the Parmesan and serve.

FRENCH GARLIC CHICKEN

You do not have to be a trained chef to make a dish that tastes like a very famous chef cooked for your family. My followers rave about this dish and the sauce has been labeled "The Sauce That Would Make a Boot Taste Good."

SERVINGS: 4

EGG-FREE
NUT-FREE
SOY-FREE

PREP TIME:
5 MINUTES

MARINATING TIME:
10 MINUTES

COOK TIME:
20 MINUTES

TOTAL TIME:
35 MINUTES

MACROS:

Fat: 65%

Carbs: 5%

Protein: 30%

PER SERVING:

Calories: 314

Total Fat: 22 g

Total Carbs: 4 g

Net Carbs: 4 g

Fiber: 0 g

Sugar: 1 g

Sugar Alcohol: 0 g

Protein: 23 g

FOR MARINATING:

2 teaspoons herbes de Provence

2 tablespoon extra-virgin olive oil

1 tablespoon Dijon mustard

1 tablespoon apple cider vinegar

½ teaspoon kosher salt

1 teaspoon black pepper

3 cloves garlic, minced

1 pound boneless, skinless chicken thighs

FOR COOKING:

2 tablespoons butter

8 cloves garlic, chopped

¼ cup heavy whipping cream

FOR MARINATING: In a medium bowl, combine the herbes de Provence, olive oil, mustard, vinegar, salt, pepper, and 3 cloves of garlic. Whisk well to emulsify the olive oil and vinegar.

Add the chicken thighs and massage to coat. Marinate at room temperature for 10 minutes or cover and refrigerate for up to 24 hours.

FOR COOKING: Heat a large heavy-bottomed skillet over medium heat; add the butter. Once the butter is melted, add the 8 cloves of chopped garlic and sauté for 2 to 3 minutes.

Add the chicken, leaving behind as much of the marinade as possible. (Do not discard the marinade.) Cook until chicken is lightly browned on one side, 3 to 5 minutes.

Add the reserved marinade and ¼ cup water. Cover and cook for 10 minutes, turning chicken once halfway through cooking time. (For safety with the marinade, the sauce must come to a complete boil while cooking, but reduce the heat as necessary to continue simmering.) Use a meat thermometer to ensure the chicken has reached an internal temperature of 165°F.

Transfer the chicken to a serving platter. Add the whipping cream to the pan and stir to combine. Bring to a simmer and cook until slightly thickened, about 5 minutes.

Pour the sauce over the chicken.

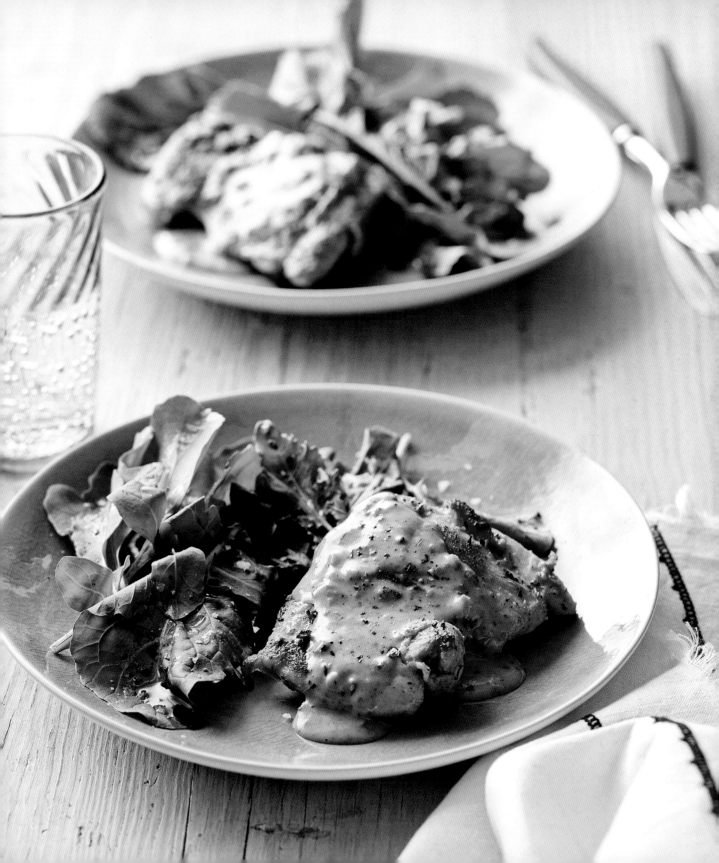

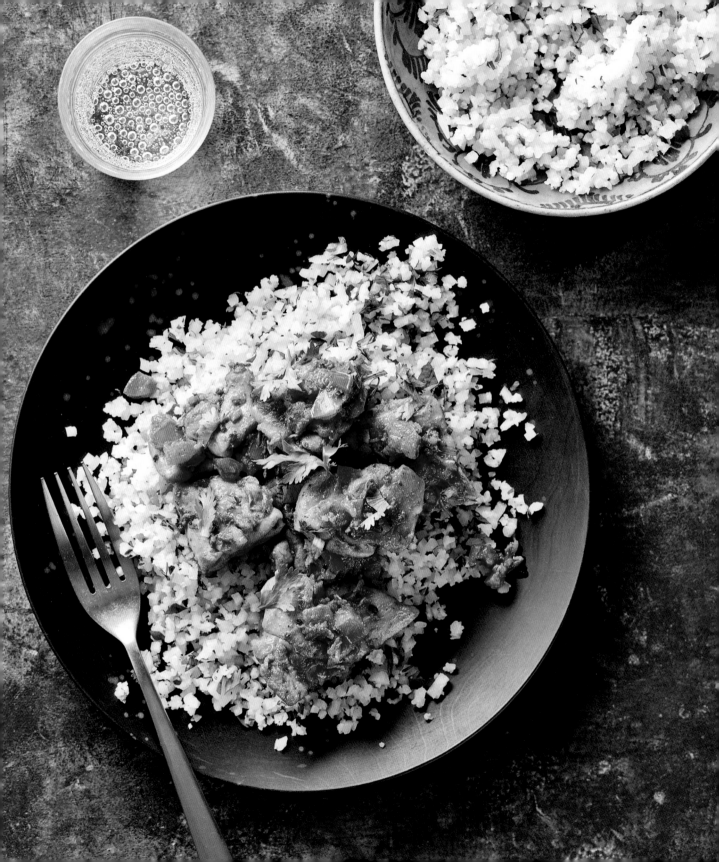

PUNJABI DRY CHICKEN CURRY

Note, the ginger is not a typo in this recipe. No really, 2 WHOLE tablespoons of it! #trustUrvashi Obviously, you'd have to love ginger to love this dish, but that's not all you taste in this recipe. It's a spicy, tomato-y, wonderful mix of flavors. Note that I cut the ginger quite small. You want to do this so you don't get a huge chunk of ginger in any one bite.

DAIRY-FREE
EGG-FREE
NUT-FREE
SOY-FREE

PREP TIME:
10 MINUTES

COOK TIME:
15 MINUTES

TOTAL TIME:
25 MINUTES

2 tablespoons vegetable oil

2 tablespoons finely diced ginger (see Note)

1 jalapeño or serrano chile, minced

1½ pounds boneless, skinless chicken thighs, each cut into 4 pieces

1 cup chopped tomatoes

2 teaspoons ground turmeric

½ teaspoon kosher salt

2 teaspoons Indian Garam Masala (page 244)

½ to 1 teaspoon cayenne pepper

2 tablespoons fresh lemon juice

¼ cup chopped fresh cilantro

HEAT a large nonstick skillet over medium-high heat; add the oil. Once the oil is hot, add the ginger and jalapeño; cook and stir for 30 seconds.

Add the chicken and sear on one side, about 1 minute; turn and sear on the other side.

Add the tomatoes, turmeric, salt, 1 teaspoon of the garam masala, and cayenne; stir to combine. Cook, uncovered, stirring occasionally, until most of the liquid has evaporated, about 10 minutes. Use a meat thermometer to ensure the chicken has reached an internal temperature of 165°F.

Sprinkle with the lemon juice, the remaining 1 teaspoon garam masala, and cilantro.

MACROS:

Fat: 45%

Carbs: 6%

Protein: 49%

PER SERVING:

Calories: 283

Total Fat: 14 g

Total Carbs: 4 g

Net Carbs: 3 g

Fiber: 1 g

Sugar: 2 g

Sugar Alcohol: 0 g

Protein: 34 g

NOTE

★ To dice the ginger, first cut it into coins. Cut the coins into matchsticks, then cut the matchsticks into dice.

SOUR CREAM SKILLET CHICKEN ENCHILADAS

Sour cream chicken enchiladas are probably a Tex-Mex invention, and they are a delicious one. There's the creamy sauce, the slight bite from the green chiles and jalapeños, hearty chicken to fill you up—oh yeah, and carby tortillas. But really, all of the flavor in this dish comes from the sauce, anyway. So why not just skip the tortillas and go straight to the sauce and chicken?

SERVINGS: 4

EGG-FREE
NUT-FREE
SOY-FREE

PREP TIME:
10 MINUTES

COOK TIME:
26 MINUTES

TOTAL TIME:
36 MINUTES

MACROS:

Fat: 61%

Carbs: 8%

Protein: 31%

PER SERVING:

Calories: 286

Total Fat: 20 g

Total Carbs: 5 g

Net Carbs: 4 g

Fiber: 1 g

Sugar: 2 g

Sugar Alcohol: 0 g

Protein: 22 g

1 tablespoon vegetable oil

4 boneless, skinless chicken thighs

½ onion, coarsely chopped

4 cloves garlic

1 (4-ounce) can diced green chiles

¼ cup chopped fresh cilantro

1 to 2 jalapeños, seeded and coarsely chopped

2 teaspoons ground cumin

1 cup shredded Monterey Jack cheese

½ cup sour cream

HEAT a large skillet over medium heat; add the oil. Once the oil is hot, add the chicken and cook for 10 minutes; turn and cook for an additional 5 minutes.

Meanwhile, in a blender or food processor, combine the onion, garlic, 1 cup water, chiles, cilantro, jalapeños, and cumin. Blend until smooth.

Pour the sauce over the chicken. Cover and cook until the chicken is tender and the internal temperature reaches 165°F, about 10 minutes.

Transfer the chicken to a serving dish. Add the cheese and sour cream to the pan and cook over low heat, stirring constantly, until the cheese is melted and the sauce is thickened, 1 to 2 minutes.

Serve the chicken with the sauce.

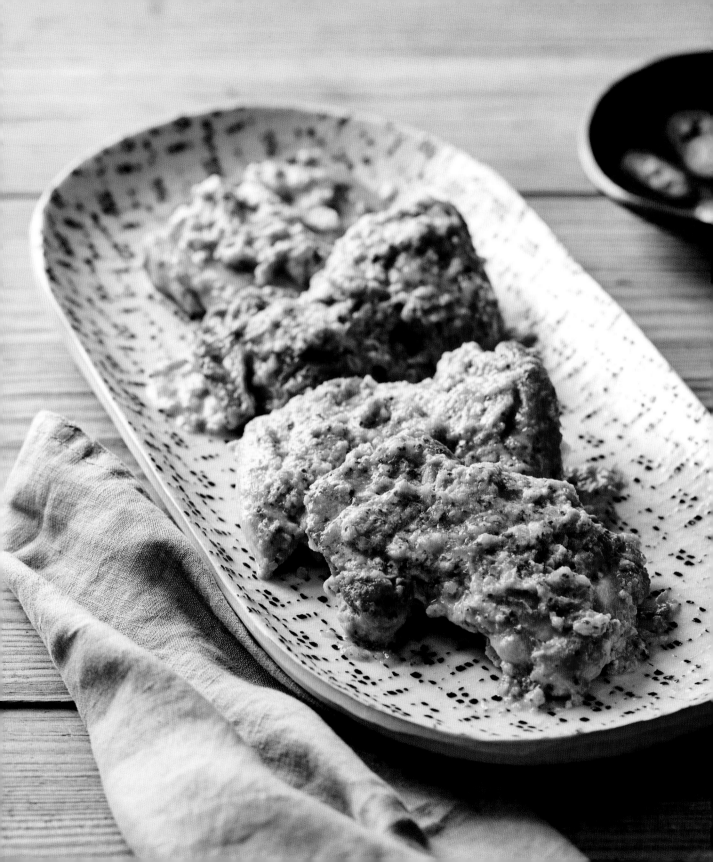

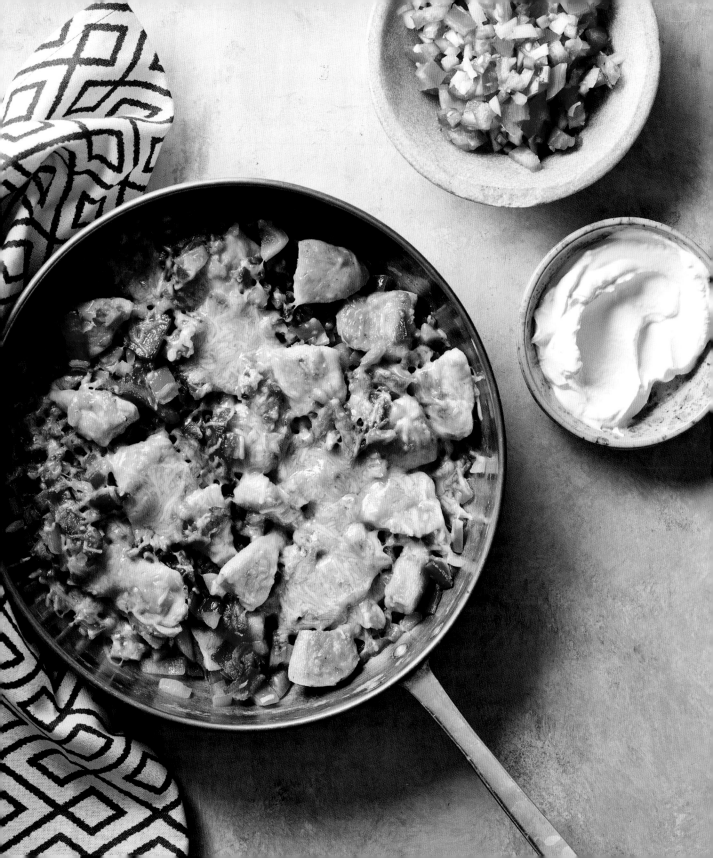

TACOS DE ALAMBRE

"Alambre" means wire in Spanish because originally the ingredients were cooked, kebab-style, skewered onto wires. There's no such time-consuming prep in this recipe. The beauty of these Tacos de Alambre is that you cook them straight in a pan, and before you know it, the well-spiced, heady mixture of chicken, veggies, chiles, and cheese sends out mouthwatering aromas that invite everyone to the table.

SERVINGS: 5

EGG-FREE
NUT-FREE
SOY-FREE

PREP TIME:
20 MINUTES

MARINATING TIME:
10 MINUTES

COOK TIME:
15 MINUTES

TOTAL TIME:
45 MINUTES

MACROS:

Fat: 53%

Carbs: 7%

Protein: 40%

PER SERVING:

Calories: 347

Total Fat: 19 g

Total Carbs: 5 g

Net Carbs: 4 g

Fiber: 1 g

Sugar: 3 g

Sugar Alcohol: 0 g

Protein: 32 g

1 pound chicken tenders, chopped

2 tablespoons fresh lime juice

1½ teaspoons kosher salt

1½ teaspoons ground cumin

1 teaspoon chili powder

6 slices bacon, chopped

½ cup chopped white onion

3 to 4 jalapeños, seeded and chopped (optional)

2 medium green bell peppers, seeded and chopped

1 cup shredded cheese (Mexican blend, Oaxaca, or muenster)

Salsa, sour cream, and/ or guacamole, for serving (optional)

IN A LARGE BOWL, combine the chicken, 1 tablespoon of the lime juice, 1 teaspoon of the salt, cumin, and chili powder. Allow to marinate at room temperature for 10 minutes.

Meanwhile, heat a large skillet on high heat. Once hot, add the bacon and cook until crisp, about 8 minutes.

Add the chicken and cook, stirring frequently, until the chicken is cooked through and no longer pink, about 4 to 5 minutes. Transfer the chicken and bacon to a bowl.

Add the onions and jalapeños, if using, to the pan. Cook until the onions are translucent, about 2 minutes. Add the bell peppers and the remaining ½ teaspoon of the salt. Cook until the peppers have softened, about 2 minutes.

Add the remaining 1 tablespoon lime juice and ¼ cup water, stirring and deglazing the pan. Add the chicken and bacon; stir to combine ingredients.

Sprinkle the cheese over the chicken and vegetables. Turn the heat to medium. Cover and allow the cheese to melt, about 2 minutes.

Serve with salsa, guacamole, and/or sour cream, if desired.

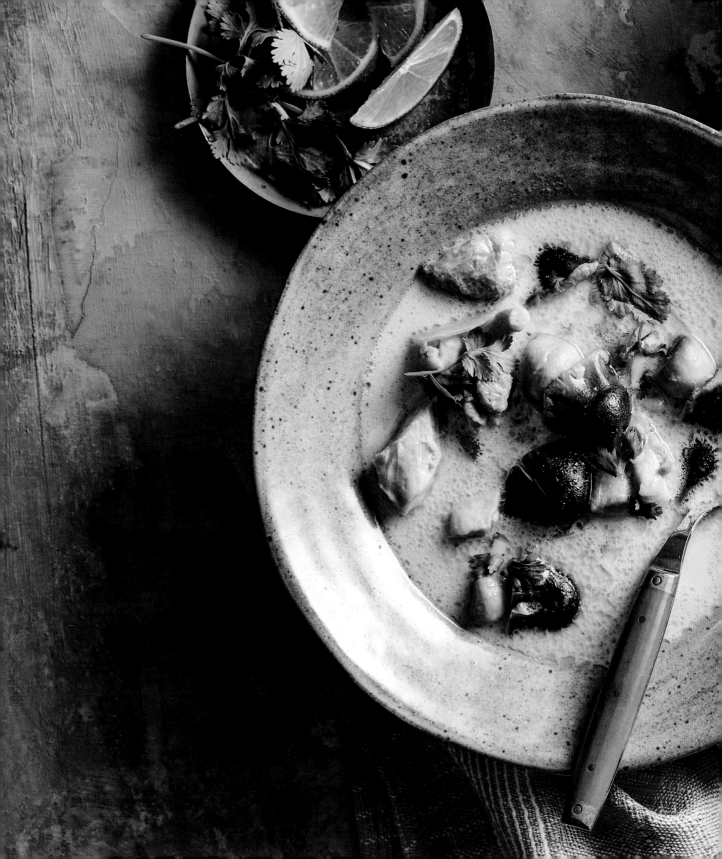

TOM KHA GAI SOUP

TOM KHA GAI SOUP

Creamy soups that are dairy-free aren't very common, but they should be. The delicate tastes of coconut milk, lemongrass, and ginger gently flavor the aromatic broth of this Thai soup—perfect for a light supper.

SERVINGS: 4

DAIRY-FREE
EGG-FREE
NUT-FREE
SOY-FREE

PREP TIME:
10 MINUTES

COOK TIME:
10 MINUTES

TOTAL TIME:
20 MINUTES

MACROS:

Fat: 52%

Carbs: 11%

Protein: 37%

PER SERVING:

Calories: 315

Total Fat: 18 g

Total Carbs: 9 g

Net Carbs: 7 g

Fiber: 1 g

Sugar: 3 g

Sugar Alcohol: 1 g

Protein: 28 g

3 cups low-sodium chicken broth

1 pound boneless skinless chicken thighs, cut into bite-size pieces

6 to 8 thin slices fresh ginger

2 whole red Thai chiles

1 cup canned straw mushrooms

2 tablespoons fish sauce

1 tablespoon minced fresh lemongrass

1 teaspoon Swerve

½ teaspoon kosher salt

1 (14-ounce) can coconut milk

Zest of 1 lime

¼ cup fresh lime juice

¼ cup chopped fresh cilantro

Lime wedges, for serving

IN A LARGE SAUCEPAN, combine the broth, chicken, ginger, chiles, mushrooms, fish sauce, lemongrass, sweetener, and salt. Bring to a boil over medium-high heat.

Lower the heat to medium and stir in the coconut milk. Simmer for 10 to 15 minutes.

Stir in the zest and lime juice.

Garnish each serving with fresh cilantro and serve with lime wedges.

SPICED CHICKEN MEATBALLS

The best way to make these North African merguez-like meatballs is—often. Actually, while that is true, what I meant to say was make the spice mix ahead of time—in fact, make two times the amount of the spice mix ahead of time, and you can put these meatballs together in no time at all. You can also use ground beef, ground lamb, or some combination.

SERVINGS: 4

DAIRY-FREE
EGG-FREE
NUT-FREE
SOY-FREE

PREP TIME:
20 MINUTES

COOK TIME:
10 MINUTES

TOTAL TIME:
30 MINUTES

MACROS:

Fat: 57%

Carbs: 4%

Protein: 39%

PER SERVING:

Calories: 204

Total Fat: 13 g

Total Carbs: 2 g

Net Carbs: 1 g

Fiber: 1 g

Sugar: 0 g

Sugar Alcohol: 0 g

Protein: 20 g

2 cloves garlic, minced

1 tablespoon sweet paprika

1 teaspoon kosher salt

1 teaspoon ground cumin

½ teaspoon black pepper

½ teaspoon ground fennel seed

½ teaspoon ground coriander

½ teaspoon cayenne pepper

¼ teaspoon allspice

1 pound ground chicken

1 tablespoon vegetable oil or extra-virgin olive oil

Tzatziki with Tahini (page 244) (optional)

Side salad (optional)

IN A SMALL BOWL, mix the garlic, paprika, salt, cumin, pepper, fennel, coriander, cayenne, and allspice until thoroughly combined.

Place the chicken in a large bowl and sprinkle the spice mix over it. Using your hands, gently mix until well combined.

Form the mixture into 16 meatballs. Heat a large skillet over medium-high heat; add the oil. Once the oil is hot, turn the heat to medium-low. Cook the meatballs until the internal temperature reaches 165°F, 10 to 12 minutes.

Serve meatballs with tzatziki, if desired, and/or a side salad.

EASY KETO CHICKEN RECIPES

There's something so efficient about buying and cooking a whole chicken, eating bits of it the first day, making bone broth with the carcass, and then continuing to repurpose it into various dishes. I give you some choices with the Chicken Cordon Bleu Casserole (page 124) and the Buffalo Chicken Casserole (page 119) but this chart has additional ideas on things that can be put together quickly with leftover cooked chicken. If you like canned chicken, you can use that. I usually just use chicken I've made in the Instant Pot or the air fryer for leftovers.

NAME	EGGS/OTHER PROTEINS	FAT	SEASONINGS/CONDIMENTS
CHICKEN TACOS WITH SALSA AND GUACAMOLE	¾ cup chopped rotisserie chicken	2 Tbsp shredded Mexican-blend or cheddar cheese Guacamole	2 Tbsp salsa Pinch each salt and pepper
CURRIED CHICKEN SALAD	1 cup chopped rotisserie chicken 1 Tbsp chopped roasted pistachios	2 Tbsp mayonnaise	2 tsp fresh lemon juice ¼ tsp curry powder Pinch each salt and pepper
CHEESY CHICKEN-BACON "RICE"	¾ cup chopped rotisserie chicken ¼ cup chicken broth 1 slice cooked and crumbled bacon	2 Tbsp cream cheese ¼ cup shredded cheddar cheese	Pinch each salt and pepper
STUFFED BELL PEPPERS	1 cup chopped rotisserie chicken	2 Tbsp cream cheese ¼ cup shredded mozzarella cheese 1 Tbsp grated Parmesan 1 Tbsp sour cream 1 Tbsp mayonnaise	Pinch each salt and pepper ¼ tsp garlic powder

VEGETABLES/HERBS	METHOD
2 butter lettuce leaves	Microwave chicken, salsa, salt, and pepper in a glass bowl for 30 to 40 seconds. Divide between lettuce leaves. Top with cheese and guacamole.
1 Tbsp minced celery 1 Tbsp minced red onion 2 tsp chopped fresh cilantro	Stir everything together.
1 cup frozen riced cauliflower	Microwave cauliflower, covered, in a glass dish for 2 minutes. Stir in chicken, broth, cream cheese, cheddar cheese, and salt and pepper. Cover and microwave for 2 minutes; stir. Top with bacon.
1 bell pepper, halved and seeded ¼ cup chopped baby spinach	Place pepper halves cut sides down in a glass dish. Cover and microwave for 3 minutes. Stir together the remaining ingredients. Divide between pepper halves. Cover and microwave until peppers are tender, 10 to 12 minutes.

EASY KETO CHICKEN RECIPES (CONTINUED)

NAME	EGGS/OTHER PROTEINS	FAT	SEASONINGS/CONDIMENTS
CHICKEN QUESADILLA	½ cup chopped rotisserie chicken	½ cup shredded Colby Jack or cheddar cheese 1 coconut-flour wrap Guacamole Sour cream	Salsa
CHICKEN NIÇOISE SALAD	¾ cup chopped rotisserie chicken 1 hard-cooked egg, halved		Vinaigrette Pinch each salt and pepper
CHICKEN "TORTILLA" SOUP	¾ cup shredded rotisserie chicken 2 cups chicken broth	2 Tbsp cream cheese ¼ cup shredded Colby or Colby Jack cheese Cheese Crisps (page 104)	2 Tbsp salsa ¼ tsp chili powder Pinch each salt and pepper
CHICKEN CAPRESE SALAD	¾ cup chopped rotisserie chicken	4 oz fresh mozzarella, sliced ¼-inch thick	1 Tbsp extra-virgin olive oil Salt and pepper
CHICKEN COUSCOUS	¾ cup chopped rotisserie chicken	1 Tbsp butter 3 Tbsp full-fat, plain, un-sweetened Greek yogurt 1 Tbsp sliced almonds	¼ tsp Ras al Hanout (page 243) Pinch of salt Harissa (page 243)
QUICK CHICKEN-FRIED RICE	1 egg, lightly beaten ¾ cup chopped rotisserie chicken		2 tsp vegetable oil 1 tsp soy sauce Pinch each salt and pepper Dash each garlic powder and onion powder 2 tsp toasted sesame oil Sesame seeds

VEGETABLES/HERBS	METHOD
	Sprinkle half of the cheese on one half of the wrap. Top with chicken. Top with remaining half of cheese. Fold over. Cook in a skillet over medium heat until wrap is browned and cheese is melted, turning once. Serve with guacamole, sour cream, and salsa.
2 Tbsp whole, pitted Kalamata or black olives ½ cup whole cooked green beans, room temperature 3 cherry tomatoes, halved	Arrange chicken, egg, olives, green beans, and tomatoes in separate piles on a plate. Drizzle with vinaigrette. Sprinkle with salt and pepper.
1 green onion, sliced	Heat chicken, broth, cream cheese, salsa, chili powder, salt, and pepper in a small saucepan over medium heat. Once hot, gradually add the shredded cheese, stirring to combine. Top with green onion and cheese crisps.
1 small tomato, sliced Handful of fresh basil leaves	Arrange the chicken, tomato slices, mozzarella slices, and basil on a plate. Drizzle with olive oil and sprinkle with salt and pepper.
1 cup frozen riced cauliflower ¼ cup frozen peas 1 green onion, sliced	Microwave cauliflower, covered, in a glass dish for 2 minutes. Stir in chicken and peas. Cover and microwave for an additional 2 minutes. Stir in the butter, ras al hanout, and salt. Top with harissa, yogurt, green onion, and almonds.
1 cup cooked riced cauliflower ¼ cup frozen peas, thawed 1 green onion, sliced	Heat vegetable oil in a small skillet over medium-high heat. When hot, cook egg until scrambled. Add the cauliflower, peas, chicken, soy sauce, salt, pepper, garlic powder, and onion powder. Cook, stirring, until heated through. Stir in sesame oil. Sprinkle with green onion and sesame seeds.

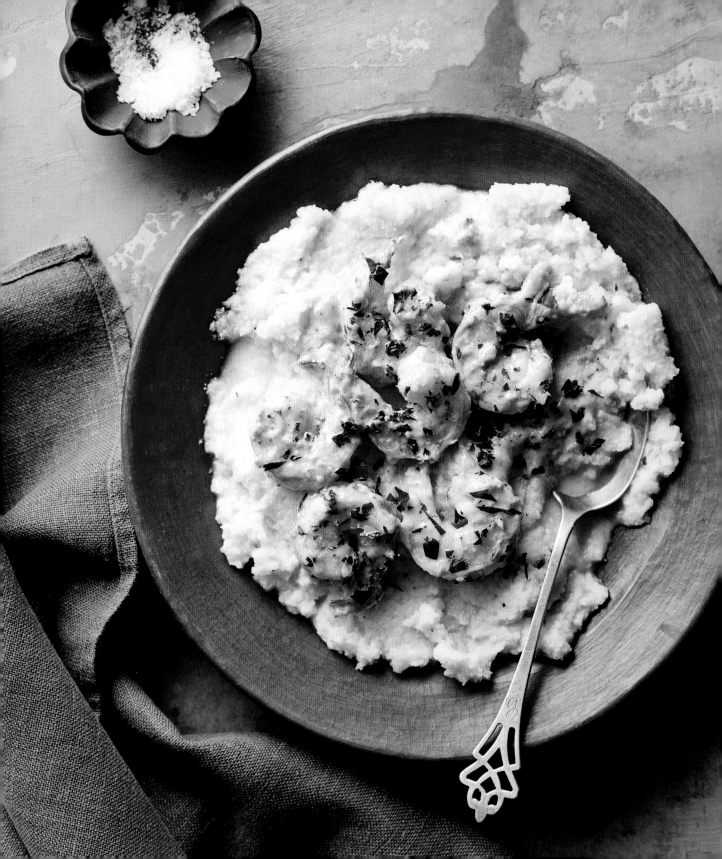

SEAFOOD

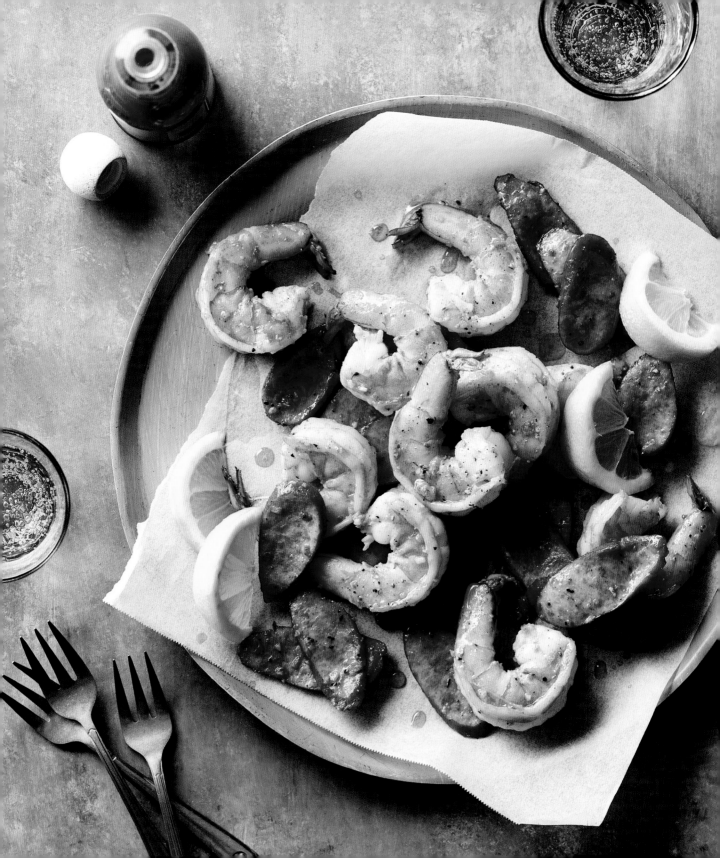

BUTTERY SAUSAGE AND SHRIMP

I mean, you had me at butter, but because I'm an overachiever, I will also give you my other favorites—sausage, shrimp, and spice. This dish tastes absolutely decadent, yet takes no time to put together. Besides, any time I have an excuse to eat melted, spiced butter straight off my plate? I'm so there!

SERVINGS: 4

EGG-FREE
NUT-FREE
SOY-FREE

PREP TIME:
5 MINUTES

COOK TIME:
5 MINUTES

TOTAL TIME:
10 MINUTES

MACROS:

Fat: 71%

Carbs: 5%

Protein: 24%

PER SERVING:

Calories: 275

Total Fat: 21 g

Total Carbs: 3 g

Net Carbs: 3 g

Fiber: 0 g

Sugar: 1 g

Sugar Alcohol: 0 g

Protein: 16 g

4 tablespoons butter

3 cloves garlic, minced

½ teaspoon paprika

⅛ teaspoon lemon pepper

⅛ teaspoon Cajun Spice (page 242)

½ pound smoked sausage, sliced

½ pound extra-large shrimp, peeled and deveined, tails removed

3 to 5 shakes hot sauce

Juice of ½ lemon

HEAT A LARGE skillet over medium heat; add the butter. When the butter is melted, stir in the garlic, paprika, lemon pepper, and cajun spice.

Add the sausage; stir to coat. Add the shrimp and cook, stirring frequently, until shrimp are pink and no longer opaque, 3 to 5 minutes. Add the hot sauce and lemon juice. Toss to coat.

Serve hot.

HOT WING SCALLOPS

Who says hot wing sauce is only for wings? Not me! I also hate asking you to buy an ingredient for just one dish. So, if you buy the hot sauce to make the Buffalo Chicken Casserole (page 119), here's an easy but tasty supper and one that looks very pretty as well. Steam some broccoli or asparagus on the side and eat up.

2 tablespoons butter

4 cloves garlic, thinly sliced

1 to 2 teaspoons hot wing sauce

1 teaspoon kosher salt

½ teaspoon paprika

1 pound bay scallops

2 tablespoons fresh lemon juice

2 tablespoons chopped fresh parsley

HEAT A LARGE saucepan over medium heat; add the butter. When the butter is melted, add the garlic, wing sauce, salt, and paprika. Simmer for 30 seconds.

Turn the heat to high. Add the scallops, turning to coat, and cook, stirring frequently, until scallops are no longer opaque, 4 to 5 minutes.

Remove from the heat. Stir in the lemon juice. Sprinkle with parsley.

SERVINGS: 4

EGG-FREE
NUT-FREE
SOY-FREE

PREP TIME:
5 MINUTES

COOK TIME:
5 MINUTES

TOTAL TIME:
10 MINUTES

MACROS:

Fat: 43%

Carbs: 16%

Protein: 41%

PER SERVING:

Calories: 137

Total Fat: 6 g

Total Carbs: 5 g

Net Carbs: 5 g

Fiber: 0 g

Sugar: 0 g

Sugar Alcohol: 0 g

Protein: 14 g

SALMON DIP

Sophisticated, smoky, creamy, and absolutely yummy, this simple salmon cream cheese dip is a crowd pleaser. Spend just $5 and have it taste like you spent about 4 times that much!

1 (6-ounce) can boneless, skinless salmon

8 ounces cream cheese, softened

1 tablespoon liquid smoke

¼ cup chopped green onions (white and green parts)

⅓ cup chopped pecans

½ teaspoon kosher salt

1 teaspoon black pepper

Paprika

Vegetable dippers, such as celery sticks, bell pepper strips, and/or broccoli and cauliflower florets (optional)

IN A LARGE BOWL, stir together the salmon, cream cheese, liquid smoke, green onion, pecans, salt, and pepper. Allow the dip to rest for 10 minutes and stir again.

Transfer to a serving bowl. Sprinkle with paprika for garnish. Serve with vegetable dippers, if desired.

VARIATIONS TO TRY

★ Substitute other nuts, such as walnuts, for the pecans.

★ Substitute sour cream for the cream cheese.

★ Add hot sauce.

★ Add Worcestershire sauce.

★ Add lemon juice.

★ Add curry powder.

★ Add chopped dill and capers.

SERVINGS: 8

EGG-FREE
SOY-FREE

PREP TIME:
10 MINUTES

STAND TIME:
10 MINUTES

TOTAL TIME:
20 MINUTES

MACROS:

Fat: 75%

Carbs: 7%

Protein: 18%

PER SERVING:

Calories: 166

Total Fat: 14 g

Total Carbs: 3 g

Net Carbs: 2 g

Fiber: 1 g

Sugar: 1 g

Sugar Alcohol: 0 g

Protein: 8 g

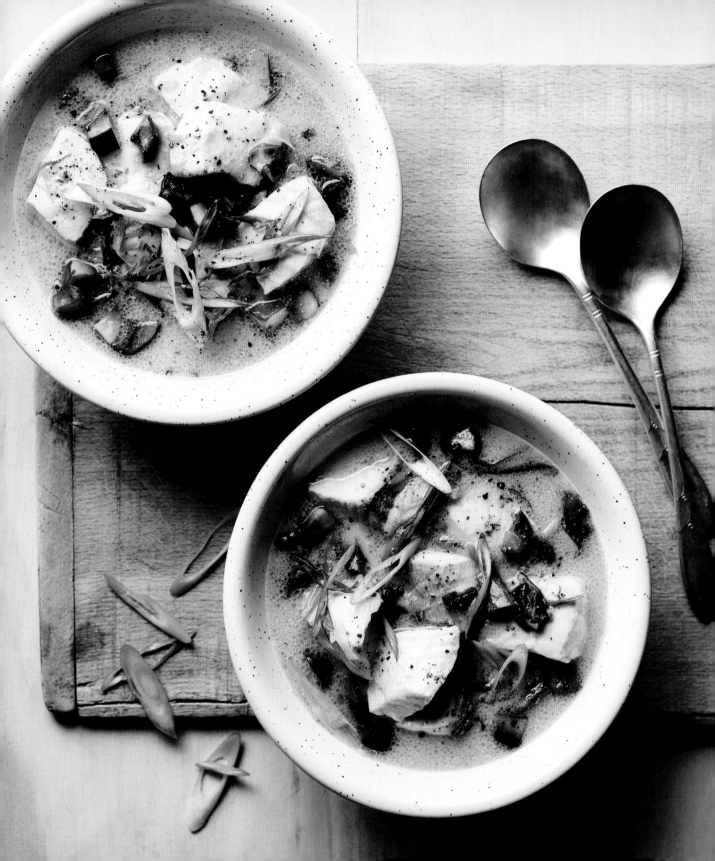

MISO SALMON CHOWDER

My friend David tested this recipe for me, and said it was so good that he would totally make it for a dinner party, but also that no one would think this was special "keto" food, which to me is what every keto recipe should be—just good food that anyone can enjoy. For those who avoid soy, use whole milk, heavy whipping cream, almond milk, or really anything else you prefer.

SERVINGS: 4

DAIRY-FREE
EGG-FREE
NUT-FREE

PREP TIME:
10 MINUTES

COOK TIME:
10 MINUTES

TOTAL TIME:
20 MINUTES

MACROS:

Fat: 50%

Carbs: 12%

Protein: 38%

PER SERVING:

Calories: 298

Total Fat: 17 g

Total Carbs: 9 g

Net Carbs: 7 g

Fiber: 2 g

Sugar: 3 g

Sugar Alcohol: 0 g

Protein: 28 g

2 tablespoons vegetable oil

¾ cup chopped green onions (white and green parts)

2 tablespoons minced fresh ginger

1 cup chopped mushrooms

2 cups unsweetened soy milk or almond milk

1 cup low-sodium chicken broth

2 tablespoons miso (white, yellow, or red)

1 teaspoon soy sauce

1 teaspoon kosher salt

1 teaspoon black pepper

½ teaspoon xanthan gum

1 pound salmon fillet, skinned and cut into bite-size chunks

1 tablespoon rice vinegar or mirin

HEAT A LARGE saucepan over high heat; add the oil. Once the oil is hot, add ½ cup of the onions and ginger; stir. Add the mushrooms and cook the vegetables until the onions are translucent, 2 to 3 minutes.

Add the soy milk, broth, miso, soy sauce, salt, pepper, and xanthan gum and bring to a boil. Add the salmon. Turn heat to medium-low and cook until the salmon is cooked through, 2 to 3 minutes.

Remove the pan from the heat. Stir in the vinegar and the remaining ¼ cup green onions.

EVEN FASTER TIP

Cut the salmon while the rest of the ingredients are cooking. Make a double batch to have the next day, but do not freeze.

PESTO SALMON WITH GARLIC SPINACH

You can make your own pesto, but I will confess to buying it so that I always have it on hand. While I've written this recipe with salmon, you can use much the same technique for any firm white fish, or even cubed chicken.

SERVINGS: 4

EGG-FREE
SOY-FREE

PREP TIME:
10 MINUTES

COOK TIME:
15 MINUTES

TOTAL TIME:
25 MINUTES

COOK TEMPERATURE:
400°F

Vegetable oil

2 tablespoons butter, melted

6 cloves garlic, thinly sliced

1 teaspoon kosher salt

1 teaspoon black pepper

2 (12-ounce) packages chopped frozen spinach, thawed

4 (5- to 6-ounce) salmon fillets

½ cup prepared pesto

1 cup cherry tomatoes

Lemon wedges

PREHEAT the oven to 400°F. Grease a 9 × 13-inch glass baking dish with vegetable oil.

In a small bowl, combine the butter, garlic, salt, and pepper. In a medium bowl, combine the spinach, tomatoes, and half of the butter mixture. Spread the spinach mixture on the bottom of the prepared dish. Place the salmon on the spinach mixture. Spread the remaining butter mixture on the salmon.

Bake until the salmon flakes with a fork, about 15 minutes. Remove the baking dish from the oven and preheat the broiler. Spread the pesto over the salmon. Broil the salmon until the pesto is warmed but not browned, about 1 minute.

Serve the salmon with spinach, tomatoes, and lemon wedges.

MACROS:

Fat: 59%

Carbs: 11%

Protein: 30%

PER SERVING:

Calories: 482

Total Fat: 30 g

Total Carbs: 13 g

Net Carbs: 10 g

Fiber: 3 g

Sugar: 2 g

Sugar Alcohol: 0 g

Protein: 35 g

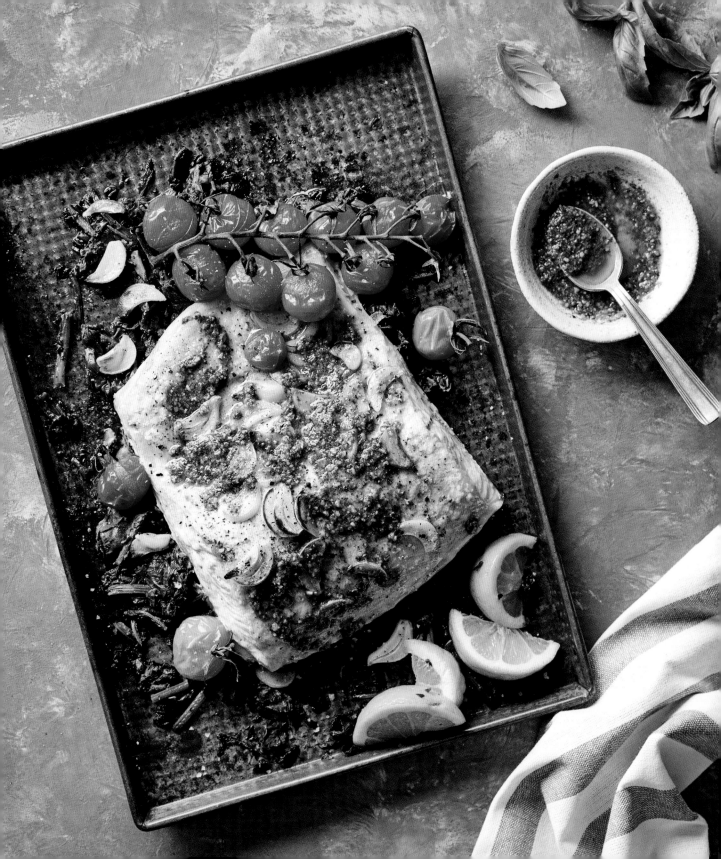

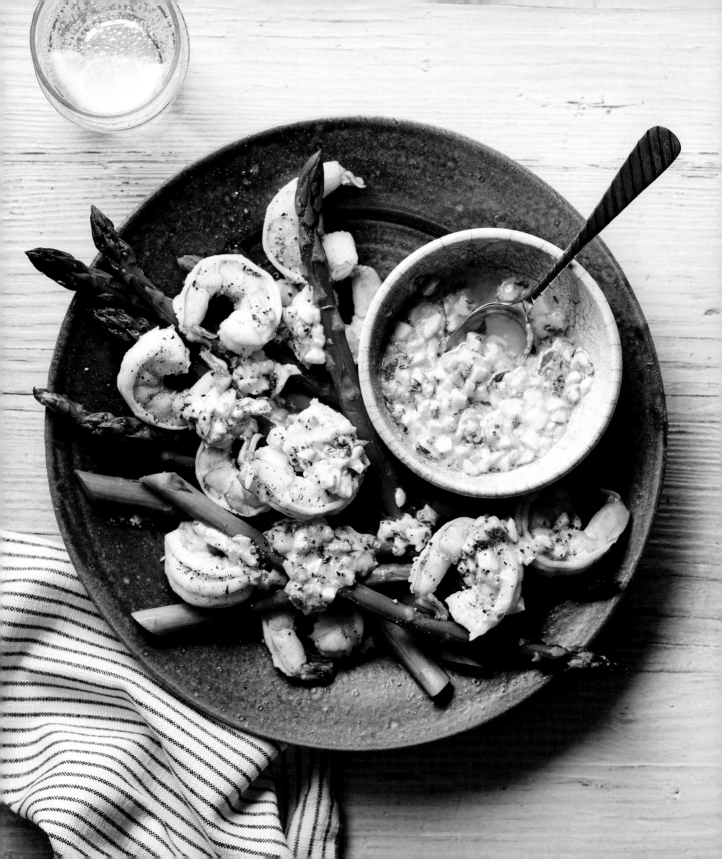

SHRIMP AND ASPARAGUS GRIBICHE

Gri-who?? Gribiche—a cold hard-boiled egg-based sauce, or another word for fat-bomb deliciousness that can be used on top of anything you please. The fact that it's made from cooked eggs makes it fast to whip together, and it also gives you yet another way to use up eggs. I've used shrimp below, but feel free to use any seafood—or even cooked chicken for this recipe. Or skip the meat entirely and make it into a vegetarian meal.

SERVINGS: 4

DAIRY-FREE
NUT-FREE
SOY-FREE

PREP TIME:
10 MINUTES

COOK TIME:
10 MINUTES

TOTAL TIME:
20 MINUTES

MACROS:

Fat: 60%

Carbs: 9%

Protein: 31%

PER SERVING:

Calories: 266

Total Fat: 18 g

Total Carbs: 6 g

Net Carbs: 4 g

Fiber: 2 g

Sugar: 2 g

Sugar Alcohol: 0 g

Protein: 21 g

1 pound shrimp (21 to 25 count), peeled and deveined, tails removed

1 pound asparagus, trimmed

2 hard-boiled large eggs, finely chopped

1 tablespoon Dijon mustard

¼ cup vegetable oil

1 tablespoon apple cider vinegar

2 to 3 tablespoons chopped dill pickles

1 tablespoon chopped fresh parsley

1 packet Splenda

½ teaspoon kosher salt

½ teaspoon black pepper

IN A LARGE SAUCEPAN, bring the 4 cups of water to a boil. Once boiling, add the shrimp and asparagus. Remove the pan from heat and cover. Let stand for 5 minutes; drain.

Meanwhile, in a small bowl, combine the eggs, mustard, oil, vinegar, pickles, parsley, sweetener, salt, and pepper.

Transfer the shrimp and asparagus to a serving platter. Pour the gribiche over and serve.

SHRIMP AND GRITS

Yeah, not really grits, but I don't think you'll care. That keto staple, the humble cauliflower, takes on yet another guise to form the perfect foil for the spicy, buttery shrimp in this recipe. I fed it to my taste testers without commenting on it, and absolutely no one complained about the lack of real grits.

SERVINGS: 4

EGG-FREE
NUT-FREE
SOY-FREE

PREP TIME:
10 MINUTES

COOK TIME:
10 MINUTES

TOTAL TIME:
20 MINUTES

MACROS:

Fat: 63%

Carbs: 11%

Protein: 26%

PER SERVING:

Calories: 335

Total Fat: 24 g

Total Carbs: 9 g

Net Carbs: 7 g

Fiber: 2 g

Sugar: 3 g

Sugar Alcohol: 0 g

Protein: 22 g

FOR THE GRITS
4 cups cauliflower florets

½ cup shredded Parmesan cheese

2 tablespoons butter

½ teaspoon kosher salt

½ teaspoon black pepper

FOR THE SHRIMP
1 tablespoon butter

3 cloves garlic, minced

1 pound shrimp (21 to 25 count), peeled and deveined, tails removed

½ cup heavy whipping cream

2 teaspoons Cajun Spice (page 242)

2 tablespoons fresh lemon juice

¼ cup chopped fresh parsley

FOR THE GRITS: In a medium saucepan, combine the cauliflower and 1 cup water. Bring to a boil over high heat. Reduce heat to medium-low. Cover and cook until cauliflower is softened, about 5 minutes; drain.

Add the Parmesan, butter, salt, and pepper. Using an immersion blender, puree until smooth. Add a little water, if needed, to thin. Cover and keep warm.

FOR THE SHRIMP: Heat a large skillet over medium-low heat; add the butter. Once the butter has melted, add the garlic and sauté for 30 seconds.

Add the shrimp, cream, and cajun spice. Cook, stirring occasionally, until the shrimp are pink and no longer opaque, about 5 minutes.

Stir in the lemon juice and parsley.

Serve the shrimp on top of the cauliflower "grits."

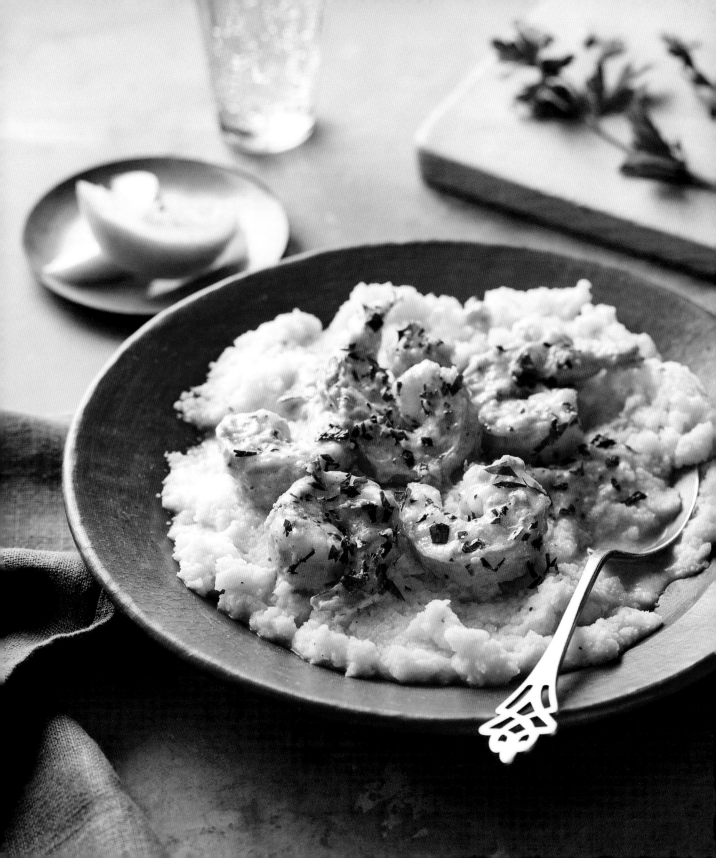

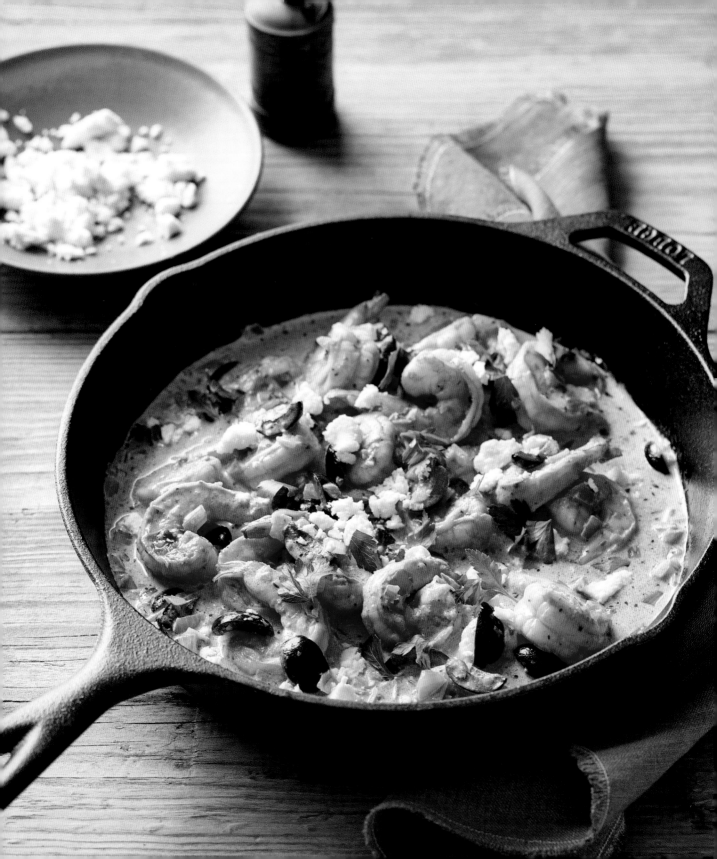

SHRIMP WITH FETA AND TOMATOES

As succulent as it is easy, this dish is also flexible enough to take on any tangy, semi-firm cheese you choose to throw at it. In fact, there's no reason you couldn't add goat cheese instead of feta, or queso fresco if you so choose. I'm not usually a fan of seafood and cheese, but this dish is an exception worth making.

SERVINGS: 6

EGG-FREE
NUT-FREE
SOY-FREE

PREP TIME:
5 MINUTES

COOK TIME:
10 MINUTES

TOTAL TIME:
15 MINUTES

MACROS:

Fat: 69%

Carbs: 10%

Protein: 20%

PER SERVING:

Calories: 298

Total Fat: 23 g

Total Carbs: 8 g

Net Carbs: 6 g

Fiber: 2 g

Sugar: 3 g

Sugar Alcohol: 0 g

Protein: 15 g

3 tablespoons butter

3 cloves garlic, minced

½ to 1 teaspoon red pepper flakes

1 cup chopped onion

1 tablespoon plus 1½ teaspoons tomato paste

1 teaspoon dried oregano

1 teaspoon black pepper

½ teaspoon kosher salt

¾ cup heavy whipping cream

1 pound shrimp (21 to 25 count), peeled and deveined, tails removed

1 cup crumbled feta cheese

½ cup sliced black olives

¼ cup chopped fresh parsley

HEAT A LARGE skillet over medium-high heat; add the butter. Once the butter is melted, add the garlic and red pepper flakes. Cook and stir for 10 to 15 seconds.

Add the onion, ¼ cup water, tomato paste, oregano, pepper, and salt. Cook and stir until the tomato paste has blended in. Cover and cook for 3 to 4 minutes.

Slowly add the cream, stirring continuously. Add the shrimp, cheese, and olives. Cook, stirring frequently, until shrimp are pink and no longer opaque, 2 to 3 minutes.

Garnish with parsley and serve.

SHRIMP WITH TOMATILLOS AND COTIJA

Tomatillos look like tomatoes, but are firmer and green in color. They have fewer net carbs than tomatoes. But mainly they have a lovely tart and tangy flavor that works really well in this dish.

1 tablespoon vegetable oil

½ cup chopped onion

2 jalapeños, seeded and minced

5 cloves garlic, thinly sliced

¾ pound fresh tomatillos, husks removed, rinsed, and chopped

1 teaspoon kosher salt

1 teaspoon black pepper

1 teaspoon ground cumin

1 pound shrimp (21 to 25 count), peeled and deveined

1 cup crumbled cotija or feta cheese

1 lime, halved

¼ cup chopped fresh cilantro

HEAT A LARGE skillet over medium-high heat; add the oil. Once the oil is hot, add the onion and jalapeños and cook until the onions are translucent, 3 to 5 minutes.

Add the garlic and stir to combine. Add the tomatillos, ¼ cup water, salt, pepper, and cumin. Cover and cook until the tomatillos are cooked but still hold their shape, 8 to 10 minutes.

Add the shrimp and cheese; stir to combine. Cook, stirring occasionally, until the shrimp are pink and no longer opaque, 5 to 6 minutes.

Squeeze the lime halves over the shrimp mixture. Sprinkle with the cilantro. Stir to combine.

SERVINGS: 4

EGG-FREE
NUT-FREE
SOY-FREE

PREP TIME:
10 MINUTES

COOK TIME:
16 MINUTES

TOTAL TIME:
26 MINUTES

MACROS:

Fat: 49%

Carbs: 17%

Protein: 34%

PER SERVING:

Calories: 269

Total Fat: 15 g

Total Carbs: 12 g

Net Carbs: 10 g

Fiber: 2 g

Sugar: 5 g

Sugar Alcohol: 0 g

Protein: 23 g

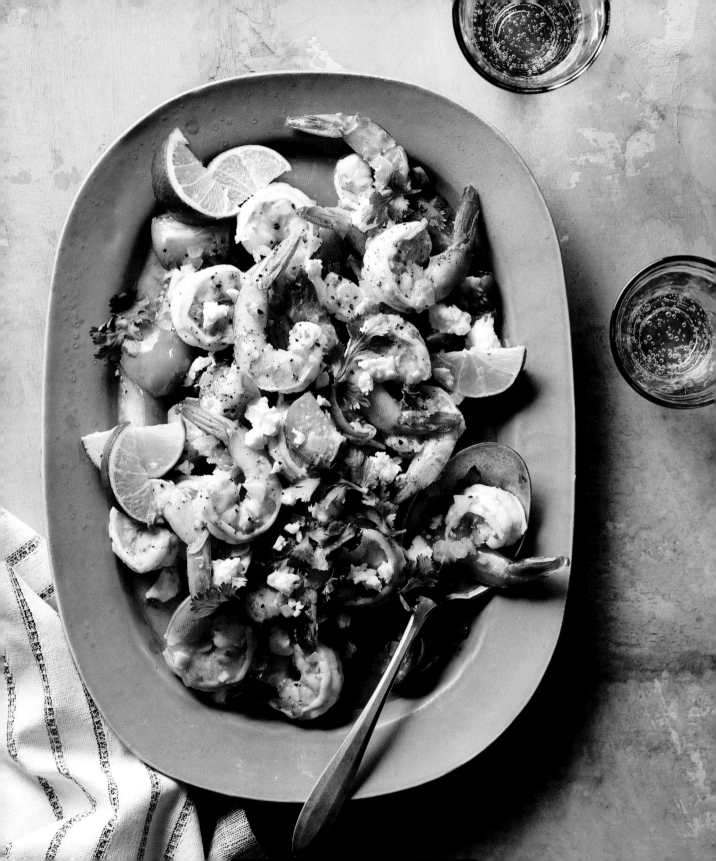

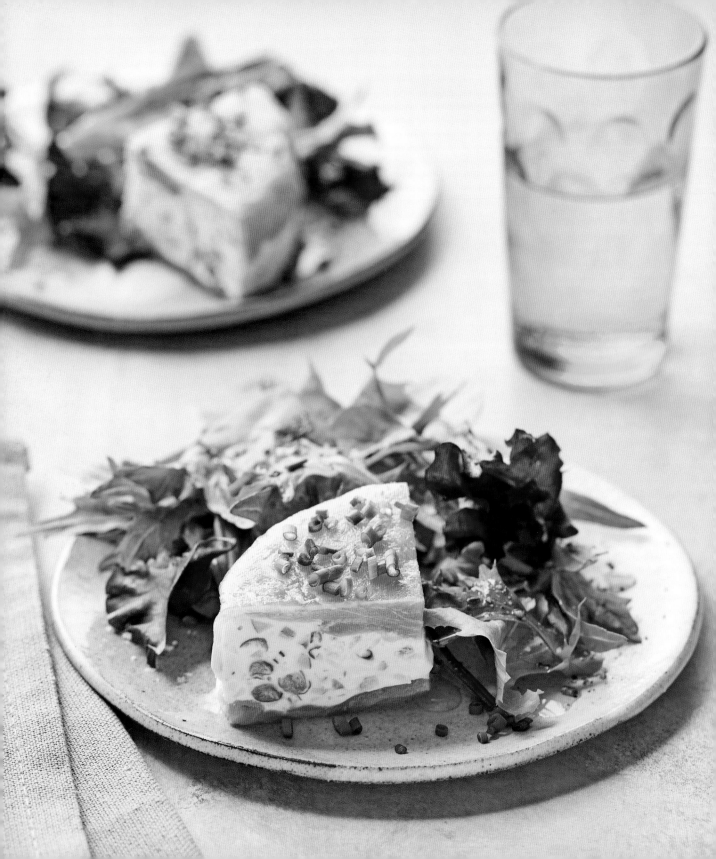

SMOKED SALMON AND CHEESE TIMBALE

This recipe is all about the elegant presentation that takes almost no time to make. By using mascarpone cheese, which is already softer than cream cheese, you shave off a little time spent standing around, waiting for cream cheese to behave. You can also use goat cheese, or a combination of mascarpone and feta for this recipe, just to change things up. When served with a side salad, you may find that the combination of cheese and salmon, filled with fat and flavor, makes quite a satisfying supper, despite its small size.

SERVINGS: 4

EGG-FREE
NUT-FREE
SOY-FREE

PREP TIME:
15 MINUTES

CHILL TIME:
10 MINUTES

TOTAL TIME:
25 MINUTES

MACROS:

Fat: 67%

Carbs: 7%

Protein: 26%

PER SERVING:

Calories: 206

Total Fat: 16 g

Total Carbs: 4 g

Net Carbs: 3 g

Fiber: 1 g

Sugar: 0 g

Sugar Alcohol: 0 g

Protein: 14 g

¼ cup finely diced red onion

4 ounces mascarpone cheese, softened

1 tablespoon fresh lemon juice

1 tablespoon capers

1 tablespoon chopped chives, plus more for garnishing

½ teaspoon kosher salt

½ teaspoon black pepper

8 ounces smoked salmon, slices cut in half the short way

6 cups spring mix salad greens

IN A MEDIUM BOWL, combine the onion, cheese, lemon juice, capers, 1 tablespoon chives, salt, and pepper. Stir until well-combined.

Line a 4-inch-wide × 2-inch-tall round baking pan with plastic wrap. Arrange 8 half-slices of the smoked salmon in the bottom of the pan. Top with the cheese mixture. Arrange the remaining 8 half-slices of smoked salmon on top of the cheese. Cover lightly with plastic wrap. Chill for 10 minutes.

To serve, unmold the timbale onto a plate. Garnish with additional chives. Cut into four wedges. Divide the greens among four serving plates. Serve timbale wedges with greens.

SPICY TUNA SALAD

This is my version of a spicy tuna roll—minus the carbs and the rolling. This method gives you the taste you crave without the work of rolling up the sushi. This makes four very generous servings. While you could have leftovers for lunch the next day, plan to eat it within 24 hours of making it. You can also make this recipe with cooked shrimp.

SERVINGS: 4

DAIRY-FREE
NUT-FREE
SOY-FREE

PREP TIME:
15 MINUTES

TOTAL TIME:
15 MINUTES

1 pound sushi-grade tuna, diced

2 cups diced cucumbers

¼ cup mayonnaise

¼ cup diced red onion

3 tablespoons fresh lemon juice

2 to 3 tablespoons sriracha

1 large ripe avocado, pitted, peeled, and diced

½ to 1 teaspoon kosher salt

1 sheet nori, cut into pieces (optional)

IN A LARGE BOWL, combine the tuna, cucumbers, mayonnaise, onion, lemon juice, sriracha, avocado, salt, and nori, if using. Stir gently to combine; serve immediately.

> NOTE
>
> ★ A mechanical chopper of some kind will speed up your prep for this recipe. Alternatively, you could pulse the ingredients in food processor to chop— but be very careful not to overprocess.

MACROS:

Fat: 50%

Carbs: 11%

Protein: 39%

PER SERVING:

Calories: 296

Total Fat: 16 g

Total Carbs: 8 g

Net Carbs: 5 g

Fiber: 3 g

Sugar: 3 g

Sugar Alcohol: 0 g

Protein: 29 g

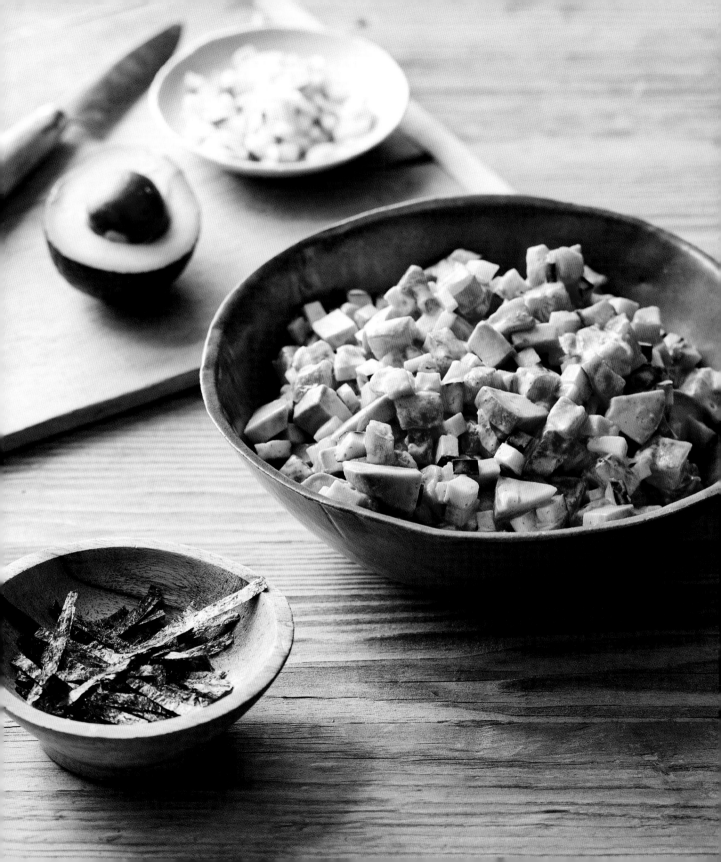

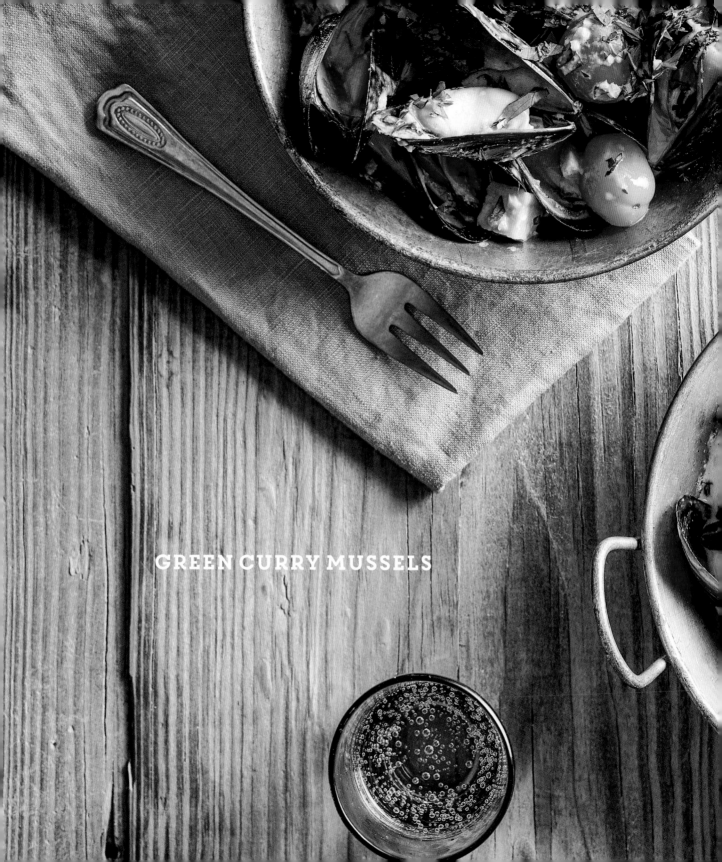

GREEN CURRY MUSSELS

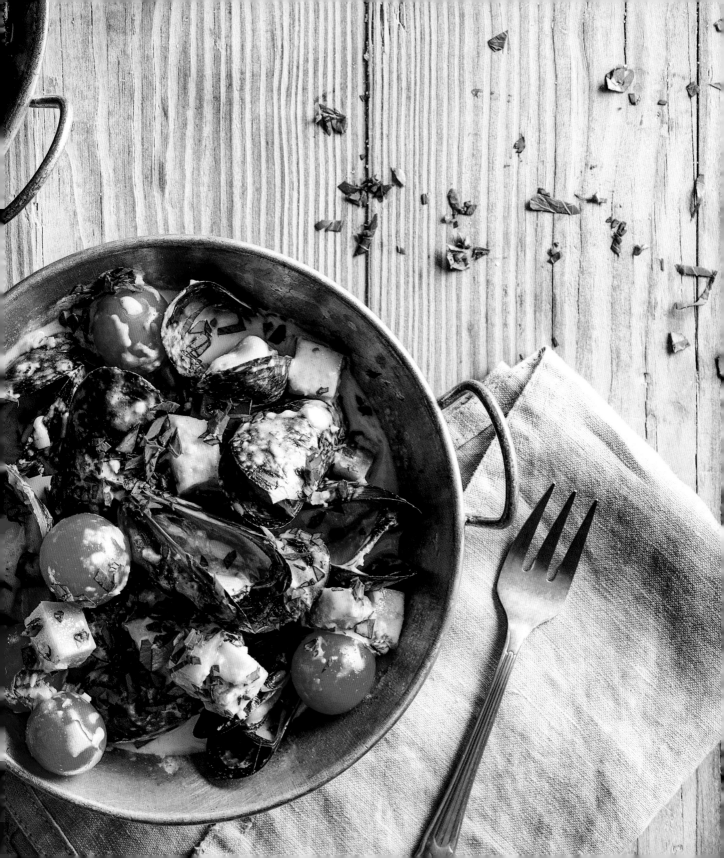

GREEN CURRY MUSSELS

I realize that mussels are not typically what we expect in Thai curries—but why not? It does make for slightly messy eating, but it also makes for very good eating. And for good food that's ready in less than 30 minutes? I'll deal with the messy.

1 tablespoon coconut oil

2 tablespoons green curry paste

1 cup chopped eggplant

½ cup cherry tomatoes

1 tablespoon minced fresh ginger

3 cloves garlic, minced

1 (14-ounce) can coconut milk

2 teaspoons soy sauce

2 teaspoons fish sauce

1 teaspoon Swerve

½ cup chopped fresh basil

1 pound mussels, scrubbed, debearded if necessary

HEAT A LARGE skillet over medium-high heat. Add the coconut oil and green curry paste. Cook and stir for 1 minute.

Add the eggplant, tomatoes, ginger, and garlic. Cook and stir for 1 minute.

Add the coconut milk, soy sauce, fish sauce, sweetener, and ¼ cup of the chopped basil. Cover and cook until the eggplant is cooked through, about 10 minutes.

Add the mussels. Cover and cook until the mussels have opened, 3 to 5 minutes. Discard any mussels that have not opened.

Stir in the remaining ¼ cup basil.

SERVINGS: 4

DAIRY-FREE
EGG-FREE
NUT-FREE

PREP TIME:
10 MINUTES

COOK TIME:
15 MINUTES

TOTAL TIME:
25 MINUTES

MACROS:

Fat: 64%

Carbs: 17%

Protein: 19%

PER SERVING:

Calories: 279

Total Fat: 19 g

Total Carbs: 12 g

Net Carbs: 10 g

Fiber: 1 g

Sugar: 4 g

Sugar Alcohol: 1 g

Protein: 13 g

SMOKY SHRIMP SCAMPI

Once again, here is a fast dish that's flexible. There's no reason you can't use clams or scallops in this sauce. It won't keep very well, so all the more reason to gobble down all of it in one dinner.

SERVINGS: 4

EGG-FREE
NUT-FREE
SOY-FREE

PREP TIME:
5 MINUTES

COOK TIME:
5 MINUTES

TOTAL TIME:
10 MINUTES

MACROS:

Fat: 61%

Carbs: 5%

Protein: 34%

PER SERVING:

Calories: 188

Total Fat: 13 g

Total Carbs: 2 g

Net Carbs: 2 g

Fiber: 0 g

Sugar: 0 g

Sugar Alcohol: 0 g

Protein: 16 g

4 tablespoons butter

3 cloves garlic, minced

1 teaspoon smoked paprika

1 teaspoon dried basil

2 tablespoons low-sodium chicken broth or white wine

1 pound shrimp (21 to 25 count), peeled and deveined

1 tablespoon fresh lemon juice

HEAT A LARGE skillet over medium-high heat. Add the butter, garlic, paprika, and basil. Cook, stirring occasionally, until the butter has melted and the ingredients are combined, about 1 minute.

Add the broth and shrimp; stir to combine. Cook until shrimp are pink and no longer opaque, 3 to 5 minutes. Push the shrimp to one side of the pan and add the lemon juice. Whisk the sauce to emulsify. Stir to coat the shrimp in sauce.

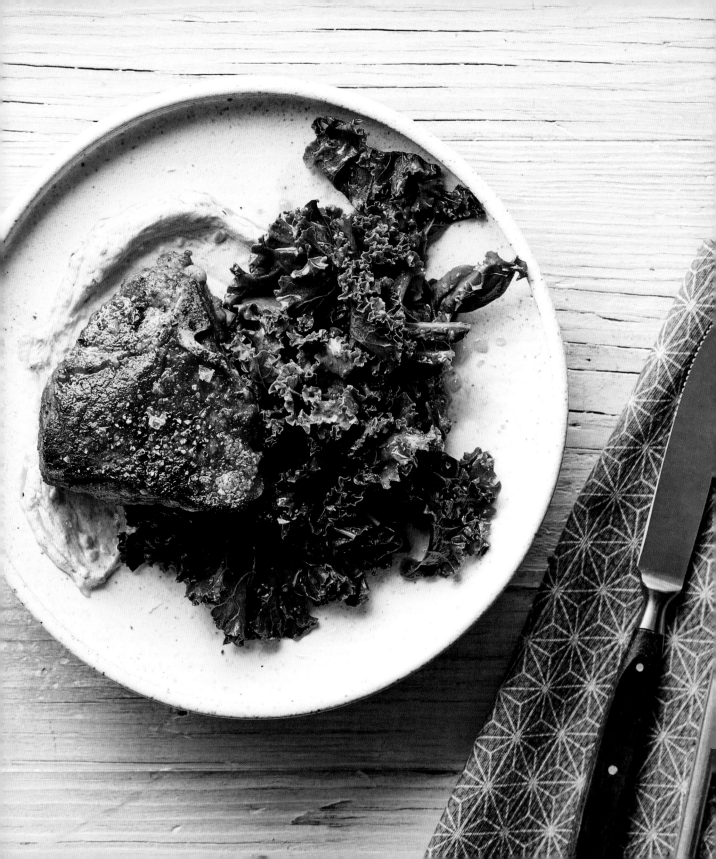

BEEF, PORK, & LAMB

BEEF SHAWARMA

True, there's no such thing as ground beef shawarma. But there is this deliciousness that tastes like a shawarma—minus all the work and time. The key to this recipe is the shawarma mix. People, it is aaaaalll about that freshly ground spice mix. In a recipe with so few ingredients, you want to amp up the taste with using the best-quality spices you can.

FOR THE SHAWARMA SPICE MIX

2 teaspoons dried oregano

1 teaspoon kosher salt

1 teaspoon ground cinnamon

1 teaspoon ground coriander

½ teaspoon ground allspice

½ teaspoon cayenne pepper

FOR THE GROUND BEEF

2 tablespoons extra-virgin olive oil

1 pound 85 percent lean ground beef

1 cup sliced onion

3 cups shredded cabbage

1 tablespoon fresh lemon juice (optional)

¼ cup chopped fresh parsley, for garnish

Tzatziki (page 244) (optional)

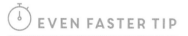 EVEN FASTER TIP

Use prepackaged coleslaw mix for the cabbage.

FOR THE SHAWARMA SPICE MIX: In a small bowl stir together the oregano, salt, cinnamon, coriander, allspice, and cayenne; set aside.

FOR THE GROUND BEEF: Heat a large skillet over medium heat; add the oil. Once the oil is hot, add the ground beef and cook, breaking it up with a wooden spoon, until almost cooked, 4 to 5 minutes.

Turn the heat to high. Add the onions and cook until translucent, 3 to 4 minutes. Add 2 tablespoons of the shawarma mix and the salt; stir well. Stir in the cabbage. Add 2 tablespoons of water and cover.

Allow the cabbage to steam for about 1 minute. Open the lid and stir well to combine. Sprinkle with lemon juice, if using.

Garnish with parsley and serve with tzatziki, if desired.

NOTES

★ This recipe freezes very well.

★ This makes 4 tablespoons of shawarma spice mix. Store in an airtight container in a cool, dark place.

SERVINGS: 4

DAIRY-FREE
EGG-FREE
NUT-FREE
SOY-FREE

PREP TIME:
10 MINUTES

COOK TIME:
15 MINUTES

TOTAL TIME:
25 MINUTES

MACROS:

Fat: 64%

Carbs: 9%

Protein: 27%

PER SERVING:

Calories: 337

Total Fat: 24 g

Total Carbs: 8 g

Net Carbs: 5 g

Fiber: 3 g

Sugar: 3 g

Sugar Alcohol: 0 g

Protein: 22 g

BEEF STROGANOFF

I ask you to remove half the onions and mushrooms and then mix them in at the end. I don't normally ask for fussy things like this, but with repeated tests, I found that you need some of that onion and mushroom flavor in the cooking—but you also need some of it at the end. It adds a nice little burst of fresh flavor that keeps the dish from tasting flat.

SERVINGS: 4

EGG-FREE
NUT-FREE
SOY-FREE

PREP TIME:
15 MINUTES

COOK TIME:
15 MINUTES

TOTAL TIME:
30 MINUTES

MACROS:

Fat: 64%

Carbs: 9%

Protein: 27%

PER SERVING:

Calories: 368

Total Fat: 26 g

Total Carbs: 9 g

Net Carbs: 7 g

Fiber: 2 g

Sugar: 5 g

Sugar Alcohol: 0 g

Protein: 24 g

1 tablespoon vegetable oil

½ cup diced onion

3 cloves garlic, minced

1½ cups chopped mushrooms

1 pound 85 percent lean ground beef

½ cup beef broth

1 tablespoon Worcestershire sauce

1 tablespoon Dijon mustard

1 teaspoon kosher salt

½ teaspoon black pepper

2 large zucchini

1 tablespoon butter

¼ cup sour cream

Cooked riced cauliflower, for serving (optional)

EVEN FASTER TIP

Buy ready-made zucchini noodles or use shirataki noodles instead.

HEAT A LARGE skillet over medium heat; add the oil. Once the oil is hot, add the onion and garlic and cook, stirring, until the onions are translucent, about 2 minutes. Add the mushrooms and cook, stirring, until softened, 1 to 2 minutes. Remove half the onion and mushroom mixture and set aside.

Add the ground beef to the skillet and cook for 2 to 3 minutes, breaking it up with a wooden spoon. Add the broth, Worcestershire sauce, mustard, salt, and pepper. Cover and cook until the beef and vegetables are cooked through, about 5 minutes.

Meanwhile, use a vegetable peeler make long ribbons from the zucchini. Place the ribbons in a microwave-safe bowl and add 2 tablespoons water. Cover and microwave on high for 2 minutes. Drain and toss with the butter.

When the ground beef is done, remove the lid and turn the heat to low. Stir in the sour cream. Simmer until mixture thickens slightly, about 5 minutes. Stir in the reserved onion and mushroom mixture.

Serve over the zucchini ribbons with cauliflower rice, if desired.

CAJUN DIRTY RICE

If you are like me, you might want a not-so-dirty variation of this by omitting the chicken livers—though chicken livers are very traditional in this classic Cajun dish. You can also use a store-bought Cajun spice mix, but if you do that, taste the dish before you add salt, as some of those prepared spice mixes contain salt. This dish reheats and also freezes very well.

SERVINGS: 4

DAIRY-FREE
EGG-FREE
NUT-FREE
SOY-FREE

PREP TIME:
10 MINUTES

COOK TIME:
15 MINUTES

TOTAL TIME:
25 MINUTES

MACROS:

Fat: 59%

Carbs: 12%

Protein: 29%

PER SERVING:

Calories: 328

Total Fat: 22 g

Total Carbs: 10 g

Net Carbs: 7 g

Fiber: 3 g

Sugar: 4 g

Sugar Alcohol: 0 g

Protein: 24 g

2 tablespoons extra-virgin olive oil

½ cup diced onion

½ cup diced celery

½ cup diced bell pepper

1 pound 85 percent lean ground beef

½ cup chopped chicken livers (optional)

1 tablespoon Cajun Spice (page 242)

2 bay leaves

2 teaspoons hot sauce

1 teaspoon kosher salt

1 teaspoon dried oregano

4 cups cauliflower rice or shredded cabbage

HEAT A LARGE skillet over medium-high heat; add the oil. Once the oil is hot, add the onion, celery, and pepper. Cook until the onions are translucent, about 1 minute.

Add the ground beef and cook for 4 to 5 minutes, breaking it up with a wooden spoon. Add the chicken livers, if using. When the beef is mostly browned, add ¼ cup water, cajun spice, bay leaves, hot sauce, salt, and oregano. Cook until the water evaporates and the spices are well incorporated into the meat, 2 to 3 minutes.

Add the cauliflower rice and cover. Cook until the cauliflower is cooked through, for an additional 1 to 2 minutes. (If using shredded cabbage, add the cabbage, cover, and remove from heat. Allow the mixture to stand for 1 to 2 minutes before serving.) Remove the bay leaves and discard.

EVEN FASTER TIP

Using a frozen, prepackaged mirepoix mix makes this a lot faster than having to dice the onions, celery, and peppers. If you can't find any frozen, dice up a double batch and freeze your own mixture for the next time you make this recipe.

EASY TACO DIP

This dip is perfect for game day, or just any day when you fancy a savory, satisfying snack. My readers love this recipe, and while many of them have made it for parties, others have it as a main dish with vegetables. You eat it the way you want to, even if it's straight out of the pot—no judging here!

SERVINGS:
6 AS AN APPETIZER, OR 4 AS A MAIN DISH

EGG-FREE
NUT-FREE
SOY-FREE

PREP TIME:
5 MINUTES

COOK TIME:
15 MINUTES

STAND TIME:
3 MINUTES

TOTAL TIME:
23 MINUTES

MACROS:

Fat: 59%

Carbs: 11%

Protein: 30%

PER SERVING:

Calories: 297

Total Fat: 19 g

Total Carbs: 8 g

Net Carbs: 7 g

Fiber: 1 g

Sugar: 3 g

Sugar Alcohol: 0 g

Protein: 22 g

1 pound 85 percent lean ground beef

½ cup chopped onion

4 cloves garlic, minced

1 (4-ounce) can diced green chiles

1 (10-ounce) can tomatoes diced tomatoes with green chiles (Ro*Tel)

3 tablespoons taco seasoning

1½ cups shredded sharp cheddar cheese

¼ cup chopped cilantro, for garnish

Raw vegetables for dipping (carrot sticks, celery sticks, radishes, cauliflower and/or broccoli florets) or cooked cauliflower rice

IN A LARGE SKILLET, combine the ground beef, onions, and garlic. Cook on medium-high heat, using a wooden spoon to break up the meat, until meat is cooked through, 5 to 6 minutes.

Add the chiles, tomatoes, and taco seasoning. Cook, stirring occasionally, until the vegetables are heated through, 5 to 6 minutes. Stir in the cheddar cheese. Remove from the heat. Cover and let stand to allow cheese to melt, 3 to 4 minutes.

Garnish with chopped cilantro. Serve with raw vegetables for dipping or with cauliflower rice.

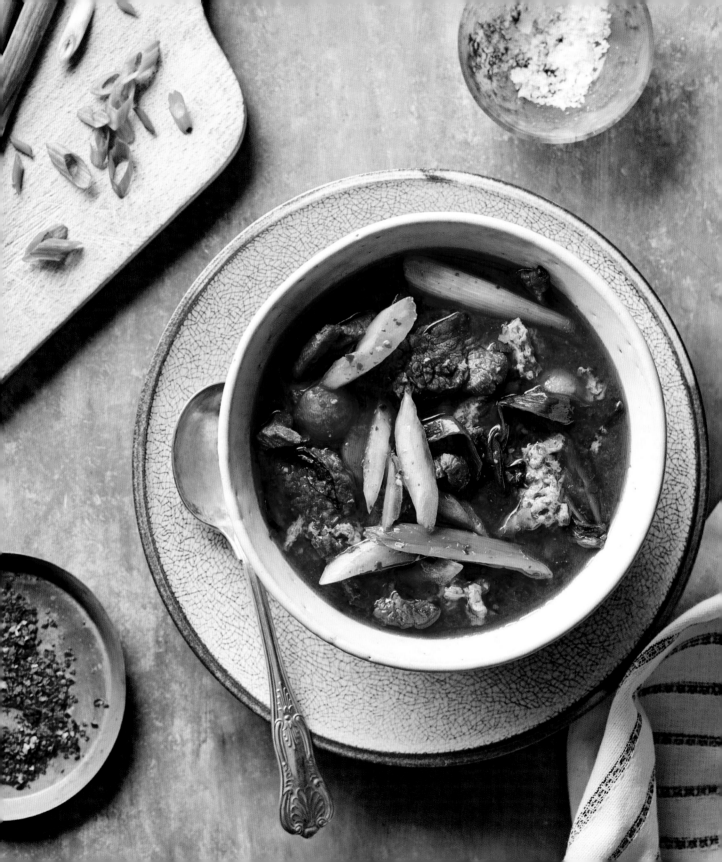

CHEATER YUKGAEJANG

Traditionally, this Korean soup is made with brisket and takes hours to make. This faster version uses flank steak. You still get the same chew and mouthfeel—but without spending hours waiting for it to cook. Spicy, meaty, and filling, don't be afraid to try this recipe. It's very approachable and will add a little zing to your meals.

SERVINGS: 6

DAIRY-FREE
NUT-FREE

PREP TIME:
15 MINUTES

COOK TIME:
15 MINUTES

TOTAL TIME:
30 MINUTES

MACROS:

Fat: 67%

Carbs: 4%

Protein: 29%

PER SERVING:

Calories: 279

Total Fat: 21 g

Total Carbs: 3 g

Net Carbs: 2 g

Fiber: 1 g

Sugar: 1 g

Sugar Alcohol: 0 g

Protein: 20 g

FOR THE PEPPER PASTE

3 tablespoons Korean hot pepper flakes (gochugaru)

3 cloves garlic, minced

2 tablespoons soy sauce

2 tablespoons sesame oil

2 tablespoons extra-virgin olive oil

2 teaspoons kosher salt

1 pound flank steak, thinly sliced on the bias

FOR THE STEW

2 cups chopped bok choy

1 bunch green onions, trimmed and cut into 2- to 3-inch pieces

1 cup radishes, cut into quarters

2 tablespoons extra-virgin olive oil

3 cups low-sodium chicken broth

2 large eggs

Pinch of salt

FOR THE PEPPER PASTE: In a medium bowl, mix together the red pepper flakes, garlic, soy sauce, sesame oil, olive oil, and salt. Transfer half the pepper paste to a large bowl. Add the flank steak to the large bowl and toss to coat; set aside.

FOR THE STEW: Add the bok choy, green onions, and radishes to the medium bowl with the remaining pepper paste; toss to coat.

Heat the oil in a large saucepan over medium-high. Once the oil is hot, add the flank steak. Cook, stirring frequently, for 2 to 3 minutes. Add the vegetables and broth.

Bring the soup to a boil. Turn the heat to medium-low. Cover and simmer for 10 minutes.

Meanwhile, beat the eggs with a pinch of salt. When the soup is done, slowly add the eggs in a steady stream to make egg flowers. Serve immediately.

> NOTE
>
> ★ This soup freezes very well and will taste even better the next day.

FLANK STEAK FAJITAS

There's something so efficient about sheet-pan dinners. There's only one pan to wash and they require minimal supervision. I like being able to make meat and veggies all together. Use colorful peppers to add some visual interest to your meal—and of course, to get a variety of nutrients in your dinner.

SERVINGS: 4

DAIRY-FREE
EGG-FREE
NUT-FREE
SOY-FREE

PREP TIME:
10 MINUTES

COOK TIME:
15 MINUTES

TOTAL TIME:
25 MINUTES

COOK TEMPERATURE:
BROIL

MACROS:

Fat: 55%

Carbs: 11%

Protein: 34%

PER SERVING:

Calories: 300

Total Fat: 19 g

Total Carbs: 8 g

Net Carbs: 6 g

Fiber: 2 g

Sugar: 4 g

Sugar Alcohol: 0 g

Protein: 25 g

FOR THE SPICE MIX

1 teaspoon ancho chile powder

½ teaspoon ground cumin

½ teaspoon ground coriander

¼ teaspoon onion powder

¼ teaspoon garlic powder

1 teaspoon kosher salt

FOR THE FAJITAS

Cooking spray

1 pound flank steak

3 tablespoons extra-virgin olive oil

2 tablespoons fresh lemon juice

1 cup coarsely chopped onion

2 cups coarsely chopped bell pepper

3 to 4 jalapeños, seeded and chopped (optional)

1 teaspoon kosher salt

FOR SERVING

Lettuce leaves (optional)

Guacamole (optional)

Shredded cheese (optional)

Sour cream (optional)

FOR THE SPICE MIX: In a small bowl, whisk together the chile powder, cumin, coriander, onion powder, garlic powder, and salt; set aside.

FOR THE FAJITAS: Place an oven rack at the highest position and turn the broiler on high. Spray a large rimmed sheet pan with nonstick cooking spray; set aside.

Place the flank steak in a large bowl. Add 2 tablespoons of the olive oil, the lemon juice, and spice mix. Massage with your hands, turning the flank steak to coat.

Arrange the onion, bell pepper, and jalapeños, if using, in a thin layer on one half of the prepared sheet pan. Pour the remaining 1 tablespoon oil over the vegetables. Sprinkle with the salt; toss to coat. Place the steak on the other side of the sheet.

Broil for 6 to 8 minutes, turning once halfway through the cook time. Check the flank steak with a thermometer (135°F for medium rare). When the steak is cooked, transfer to a plate. Cover and allow to rest for 10 minutes.

Meanwhile, toss the vegetables with tongs and broil for an additional 2 to 3 minutes. Transfer the vegetables to a serving dish.

Thinly slice the meat against the grain. Serve the meat and vegetables by themselves, or wrapped in lettuce leaves. Serve with guacamole, cheese, and/or sour cream, if desired.

VARIATIONS TO TRY

★ Turn this, or the left-overs, into a salad by adding a small amount of the spice rub to a mix of equal parts of mayo and sour cream for a dressing.

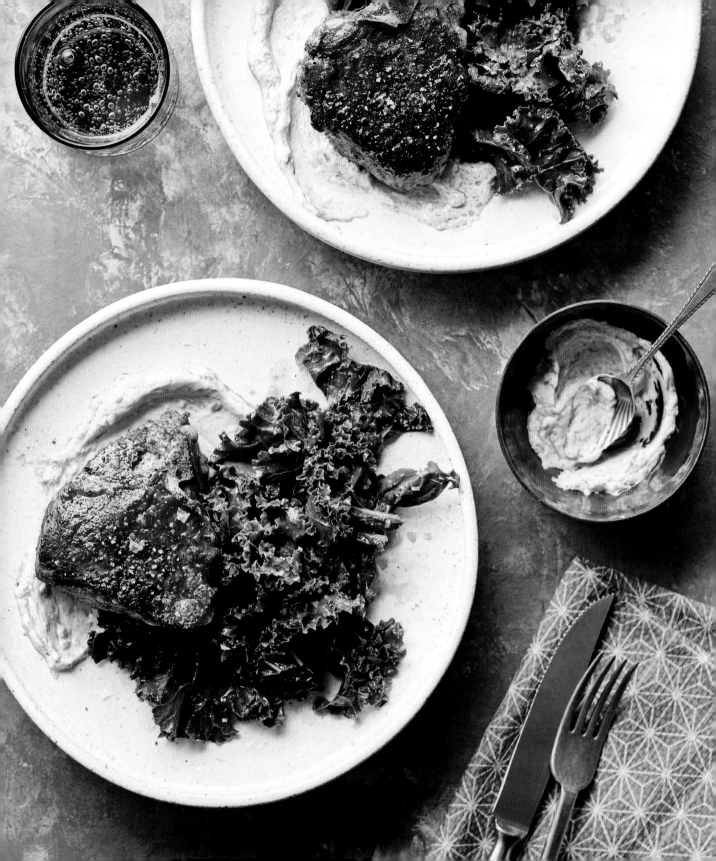

HARISSA LAMB CHOPS AND KALE

This recipe was tested using the harissa paste in this book. If you use commercially prepared harissa, you may or may not get the same burst of flavor, but I'd say make the harissa at home. Once you make it, you can use it for this as well as the Harissa-Roasted Turnips (page 89)—and it lasts for months in your fridge. You can use it for marinating meat, roasting vegetables, or as a sauce. In this recipe, that ingredient does triple duty for marinade, cooking sauce, and drizzling sauce. Because #ruthlesseffiency.

SERVINGS: 2

EGG-FREE
NUT-FREE
SOY-FREE

PREP TIME:
5 MINUTES

COOK TIME:
15 MINUTES

TOTAL TIME:
20 MINUTES

MACROS:

Fat: 67%

Carbs: 9%

Protein: 24%

PER SERVING:

Calories: 502

Total Fat: 38 g

Total Carbs: 11 g

Net Carbs: 7 g

Fiber: 4 g

Sugar: 2 g

Sugar Alcohol: 0 g

Protein: 31 g

2 loin lamb chops (5 to 6 ounces each)

3 tablespoons Harissa (page 243)

1 (10-ounce) package frozen chopped kale, thawed

½ cup sour cream

Salt

⏱ EVEN FASTER TIP

I hate washing dishes unnecessarily, so I didn't remove the lamb chops before adding the kale. It works equally well to just push them to one side, mix up the kale, put them on top of it, and proceed as directed.

IN A SMALL BOWL, coat the lamb chops with 1 tablespoon of the harissa.

Heat a large nonstick skillet over medium-high heat. Once the pan is hot, add the lamb chops. Cook on one side until a crust has formed, about 3 minutes. Turn and cook for an additional 3 minutes. Transfer to a plate.

Add the kale and ½ cup water to the saucepan and mix well, stirring to deglaze the pan. Transfer the lamb chops back to the saucepan. Cover, reduce heat to medium-low, and cook for 4 to 6 minutes. Use a meat thermometer to ensure the lamb has reached an internal temperature of 145°F (medium-rare).

Meanwhile, in a small bowl, combine the remaining 2 tablespoons of the harissa and the sour cream.

Transfer the lamb chops to serving plates.

Add half of the sour cream mixture to the saucepan; mix well. Season to taste with salt.

Drizzle the remaining sauce over the lamb chops. Serve chops with kale.

ITALIAN SAUSAGE AND SPINACH SOUP

I have never had the famous Zuppa Toscana people rave about, mainly because we rarely eat out, but also because of the potatoes in the soup. But I made this version and found that it was very well received, it comes together with very little prep time, it eats like a meal—and it freezes well. In fact, it tastes even better the next day. This makes a generous 3-quart batch, or 12 cups. I used spinach in mine, but feel free to substitute frozen kale instead. You can also use fresh spinach or kale, but you will likely need a larger pot to hold all the fresh greens.

SERVINGS: 6

EGG-FREE
NUT-FREE
SOY-FREE

PREP TIME:
15 MINUTES

COOK TIME:
15 MINUTES

TOTAL TIME:
30 MINUTES

MACROS:

Fat: 72%

Carbs: 10%

Protein: 18%

PER SERVING:

Calories: 424

Total Fat: 33 g

Total Carbs: 10 g

Net Carbs: 7 g

Fiber: 3 g

Sugar: 2 g

Sugar Alcohol: 0 g

Protein: 18 g

2 tablespoons extra-virgin olive oil

1 pound bulk hot Italian sausage

1 cup diced onion

3 cloves garlic, minced

1 (12-ounce) package frozen riced cauliflower, thawed

1 (12-ounce) package chopped frozen spinach, thawed

4 cups chicken broth

½ cup heavy whipping cream

½ cup shredded Parmesan cheese, plus more for garnish

2 teaspoons black pepper

1½ teaspoons kosher salt

HEAT A LARGE saucepan on medium-high heat; add the oil. Once hot, add the sausage and cook, breaking up the meat with a wooden spoon, until sausage is browned, 5 to 6 minutes.

Add the onion, garlic, cauliflower, spinach, and broth. Stir to combine. Cover and bring to a boil. Reduce heat and cook for 2 to 3 minutes.

Add the cream and the ½ cup Parmesan cheese. Heat to a simmer, stirring occasionally, until heated through and cheese is melted, 3 to 4 minutes. Stir in the pepper and salt.

Serve with additional cheese, if desired.

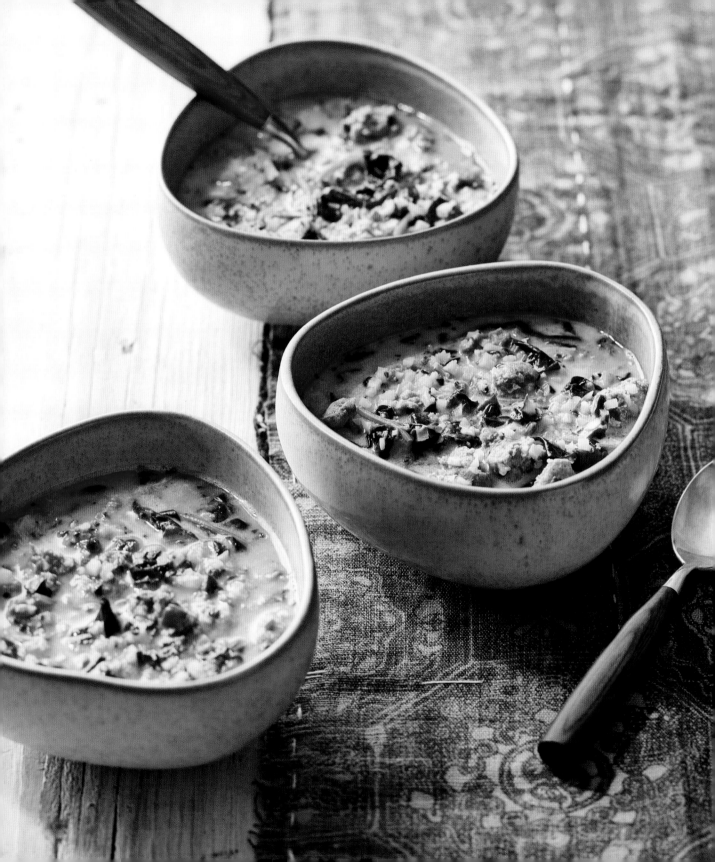

LAMB AVGOLEMONO

Fair warning, this is for serious lamb lovers. The dish is very lamby—more so than say, the Harissa Lamb Chops and Kale (page 000). But if you love lamb, then this delicately spiced, lemony lamb stew is a delight. It doesn't look like much, but it's a great, hearty, and fast supper dish. You can also make this with ground chicken if you'd prefer.

SERVINGS: 4

DAIRY-FREE
NUT-FREE
SOY-FREE

PREP TIME:
10 MINUTES

COOK TIME:
14 MINUTES

STAND TIME:
1 MINUTE

TOTAL TIME:
25 MINUTES

MACROS:

Fat: 68%

Carbs: 5%

Protein: 27%

PER SERVING:

Calories: 385

Total Fat: 28 g

Total Carbs: 5 g

Net Carbs: 4 g

Fiber: 1 g

Sugar: 1 g

Sugar Alcohol: 0 g

Protein: 25 g

1 tablespoon extra-virgin olive oil

1 pound ground lamb

½ cup diced onion

3 cloves garlic, minced

1 teaspoon dried oregano

1½ teaspoons kosher salt

1 (10-ounce) package chopped frozen spinach, thawed, or 4 cups fresh spinach leaves, chopped

2 tablespoons chopped fresh mint (optional)

¾ cup low-sodium chicken broth or water

3 large eggs, beaten

2 tablespoons fresh lemon juice

HEAT A LARGE saucepan over high heat; add the oil. Once the oil is hot, add the lamb, onion, and garlic to the pan and cook, using a wooden spoon to break up the meat, until it is no longer pink, 5 to 6 minutes. Add the oregano, salt, spinach, and broth. Reduce the heat to medium-low. Cover and cook for 5 to 6 minutes.

Meanwhile, in a small bowl, whisk together the eggs and lemon juice.

At the end of the cooking time, slowly whisk in a couple of ladles of the hot lamb mixture into the egg mixture, stirring constantly. (You are doing this to temper your eggs so they don't curdle as you pour them into the hot lamb mixture.) Slowly pour the egg mixture into the lamb, stirring constantly. Shake the pan from side to side to ensure the egg sauce has spread out over the lamb. Sprinkle with chopped mint, if using.

Turn off the heat. Cover and let stand for 1 to 2 minutes. (This allows the sauce to thicken.) Serve hot.

LEBANESE HASHWEH

A staple in Middle Eastern cuisine, *hashweh* is a flavor-packed dish made of ground meat cooked in ghee, then seasoned with cinnamon and toasted pine nuts. I typically like to make mine with cauliflower rice to add a little body to the dish.

SERVINGS: 4

DAIRY-FREE
EGG-FREE
SOY-FREE

PREP TIME:
10 MINUTES

COOK TIME:
8 MINUTES

TOTAL TIME:
18 MINUTES

MACROS:

Fat: 65%

Carbs: 11%

Protein: 24%

PER SERVING:

Calories: 391

Total Fat: 28 g

Total Carbs: 11 g

Net Carbs: 8 g

Fiber: 3 g

Sugar: 4 g

Sugar Alcohol: 0 g

Protein: 24 g

2 tablespoons Homemade Ghee (page 239), ghee, or extra-virgin olive oil

¼ cup pine nuts

1 cup sliced onion

3 cloves garlic, minced

1 pound 85 percent lean ground beef

¼ teaspoon ground cardamom

1½ teaspoons ground allspice

1 teaspoon ground cinnamon

¼ ground nutmeg

1 teaspoon kosher salt

1 teaspoon black pepper

4 cups shredded cabbage or cauliflower rice

¼ cup chopped fresh cilantro, parsley, or mint (or a mix)

HEAT A LARGE skillet over medium heat; add the ghee. Once the ghee has melted, add the pine nuts and cook, stirring for 1 to 2 minutes.

Add the onion and garlic. Cook and stir for 1 to 2 minutes. Add the ground beef and cook, breaking the meat up with a wooden spoon, for 1 to 2 minutes. Add the cardamom, allspice, cinnamon, nutmeg, salt, and pepper. Continue cooking and stirring until the beef is cooked through, 4 to 5 minutes.

Remove from the heat and stir in the shredded cabbage. Garnish with the herbs and serve.

VARIATIONS TO TRY

★ Substitute any type of nut for the pine nuts.

⏱ EVEN FASTER TIP

Double the spice mix and use it within the next 2 to 3 weeks.

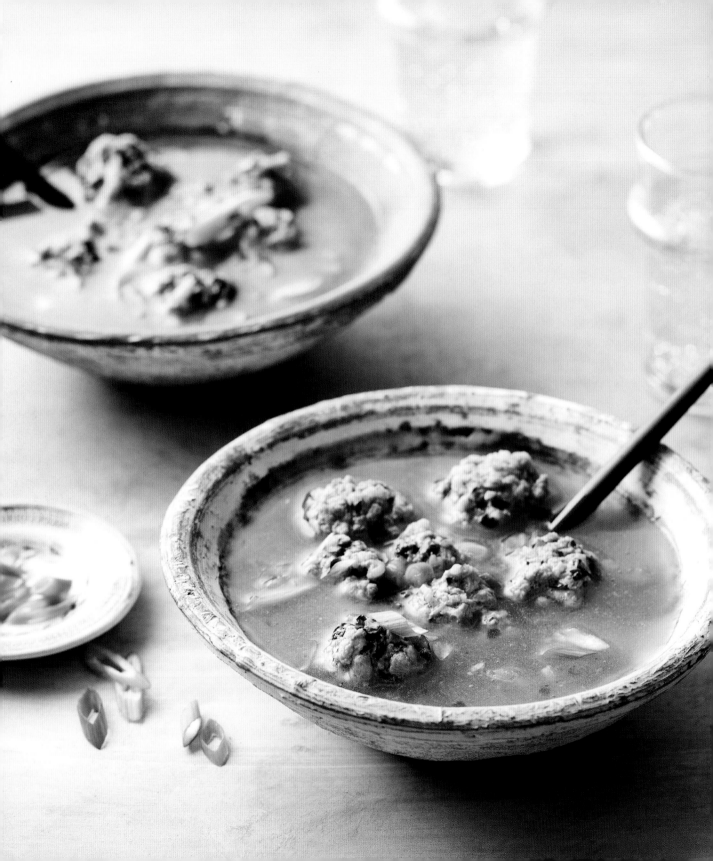

NAKED WONTON SOUP

All of the flavor of wontons, none of the work, and none of the carbs. Now that's a hard combination to beat! You can also freeze some of these wontons and just add them to broth to cook at a later date if you prefer. Add bok choy or mushrooms for a heartier soup.

SERVINGS: 4

DAIRY-FREE
NUT-FREE

PREP TIME:
15 MINUTES

COOK TIME:
10 MINUTES

TOTAL TIME:
25 MINUTES

MACROS:

Fat: 71%

Carbs: 3%

Protein: 26%

PER SERVING:

Calories: 373

Total Fat: 29 g

Total Carbs: 2 g

Net Carbs: 2 g

Fiber: 0 g

Sugar: 0 g

Sugar Alcohol: 0 g

Protein: 24 g

FOR THE BROTH

4 cups low-sodium chicken broth

1 tablespoon soy sauce

1 tablespoon sesame oil

FOR THE WONTONS

1 pound ground pork

¼ cup chopped green onions (green and white parts)

¼ cup chopped fresh cilantro or parsley

2 teaspoons soy sauce

1 tablespoon minced fresh ginger

½ teaspoon kosher salt

1 teaspoon black pepper

3 cloves garlic, minced

2 large eggs, lightly beaten

FOR THE BROTH: In a large saucepan, heat the broth, soy sauce, and sesame oil over medium-high heat.

FOR THE WONTONS: Meanwhile, in a large bowl gently mix together the pork, green onions, cilantro, soy sauce, ginger, salt, pepper, garlic, and eggs. (Keep the mixture loose—don't overwork it or your wontons will be tough.)

Once the broth has begun to boil, turn down the heat to a simmer. Using a small scoop or melon baller, scoop the pork mixture into meatballs and drop into the simmering broth. Continue until all the meat has been used up.

Bring the soup to a boil and cook until the meatballs are cooked through, 4 to 5 minutes. Use a meat thermometer to ensure the meatballs have reached an internal temperature of 160°F.

EVEN FASTER TIP

Make a double batch of the pork mixture. Freeze the other half of it in bulk, or form into meatballs and bake in a 400°F oven for 15 to 20 minutes, then freeze so you can make the soup even faster the next time.

PORK BELLY CABBAGE SOUP

This soup is creamy but dairy-free, thanks to the pork belly and miso. You can use any type of miso you have—white, yellow, or red. I know the purists might disagree with me and want me to recommend a particular type of miso, but for me, any miso is better than no miso!

SERVINGS: 4

DAIRY-FREE
EGG-FREE
NUT-FREE

PREP TIME:
5 MINUTES

COOK TIME:
15 MINUTES

TOTAL TIME:
20 MINUTES

MACROS:

Fat: 85%

Carbs: 5%

Protein: 9%

PER SERVING:

Calories: 659

Total Fat: 62 g

Total Carbs: 9 g

Net Carbs: 7 g

Fiber: 2 g

Sugar: 4 g

Sugar Alcohol: 0 g

Protein: 15 g

1 pound pork belly, cut into bite-size pieces

3 cups shredded napa cabbage

1 cup sliced mushrooms

4 cups low-sodium chicken broth

3 tablespoons miso paste (white, yellow, or red)

2 tablespoons tahini

1 teaspoon apple cider vinegar

HEAT A LARGE saucepan over high heat. When hot, add the pork belly, then immediately turn the heat to medium. (This allows the pork belly to gently render some fat.) Cook, stirring occasionally, until the meat is cooked through, about 5 minutes.

Remove all but about 2 tablespoons of the fat from the pan. Add the cabbage and mushrooms and stir until vegetables are coated with the fat.

Add the broth, miso, and tahini. Stir to combine. When the broth comes to a boil, remove the pan from the heat. Stir in the vinegar and serve.

⏱ EVEN FASTER TIPS

Double the pork belly and remove half for snacking when it has finished cooking.

Slice the vegetables as the pork belly cooks.

Buy presliced mushrooms and preshredded cabbage.

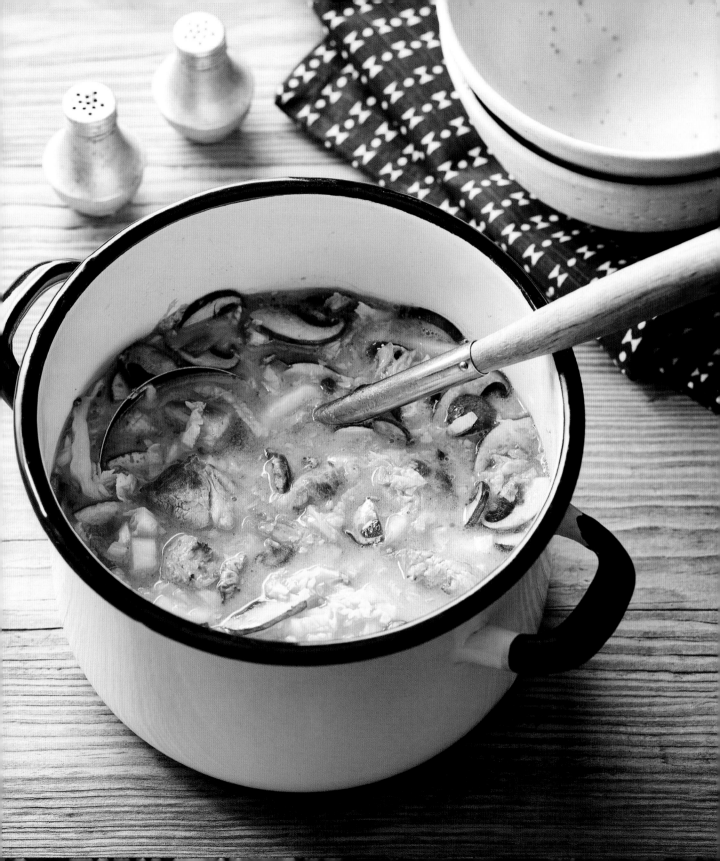

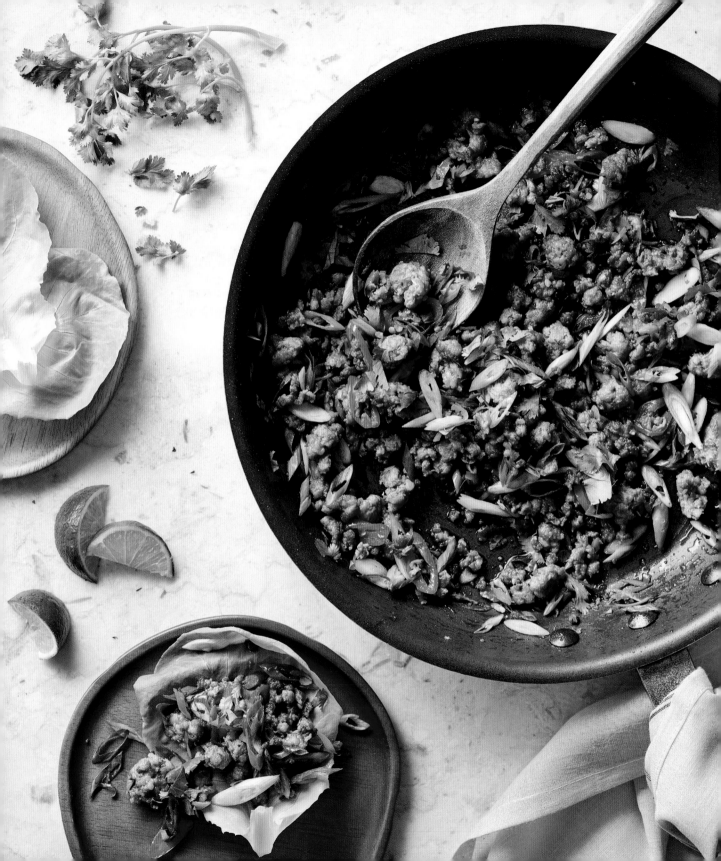

PORK CHILE LETTUCE CUPS

A little ground meat, some cilantro and chiles, a few minutes of work, and a great dinner. This will beat any of the overly sugared minced meat-and-lettuce cups at restaurants, and you won't worry about being knocked out of ketosis. Use whatever ground meat you prefer for this dish.

SERVINGS: 4

DAIRY-FREE
EGG-FREE
NUT-FREE

PREP TIME:
5 MINUTES

COOK TIME:
15 MINUTES

TOTAL TIME:
20 MINUTES

MACROS:

Fat: 76%

Carbs: 3%

Protein: 21%

PER SERVING:

Calories: 396

Total Fat: 33 g

Total Carbs: 3 g

Net Carbs: 2 g

Fiber: 1 g

Sugar: 1 g

Sugar Alcohol: 0 g

Protein: 20 g

1 tablespoon extra-virgin olive oil

1 tablespoon minced fresh ginger

3 cloves garlic, minced

1 pound ground pork

2 to 3 red and/or green chiles, sliced (such as jalapeños, serranos, or Thai bird's-eye chiles), stemmed and sliced

1 tablespoon soy sauce

2 tablespoons sesame oil

2 teaspoons sambal oelek or other spicy red chili sauce (optional)

½ cup chopped green onions

½ cup chopped fresh cilantro

1 tablespoon fresh lemon juice, or 1 tablespoon fresh lime juice

4 large lettuce leaves

HEAT A LARGE skillet over medium heat; add the olive oil. Once the oil is hot, add the ginger and garlic; cook and stir for 2 to 3 seconds. Add the ground pork and cook, breaking up the meat with a wooden spoon, until meat is browned and slightly crispy, 6 to 7 minutes.

When the pork is almost done, make a space in the middle of the pan. Add the chiles, soy sauce, sesame oil, and the sambal oelek, if using. Stir well to combine.

Remove meat off the heat and allow to cool for 3 to 4 minutes.

Stir in the green onions, cilantro, and lemon or lime juice.

Divide the meat among the lettuce leaves and serve.

PORK CHOPS AND CABBAGE WITH MUSTARD CREAM SAUCE

Mustard cream has to be a classic sauce, even for those of us (myself included) who aren't great mustard fans. In my view, a good mustard sauce has tang, but you shouldn't just taste mustard. This is an easy way to get pork chops and cabbage on the table in a hurry and that cream sauce just makes it all decadent and juicy.

4 thin center-cut boneless pork chops

1½ teaspoons kosher salt

1½ teaspoons black pepper

3 tablespoons extra-virgin olive oil

½ cup chopped onion

4 cups chopped green cabbage

1 tablespoon butter

¾ cup heavy whipping cream

2 tablespoons Dijon mustard

2 tablespoons fresh lemon juice

SEASON THE PORK CHOPS with 1 teaspoon of the salt and 1 teaspoon of the pepper.

Heat a large skillet over medium-high heat; add 1 tablespoon of the oil. Once the oil is hot, add the pork chops.

Cook until fully browned on one side, about 4 minutes. Turn and cook until the other side is browned, 2 to 3 minutes. Transfer the pork chops to a serving plate. Cover the pork chops with foil and set aside.

Add the onion to the pan and stir. Cook until the onion is translucent, 2 to 3 minutes. Stir in the cabbage. Add the remaining salt and pepper. Cook until the cabbage is tender, 2 to 3 minutes. Add the butter and toss; transfer to a serving plate.

Add the cream and mustard to the pan; stir until the mustard is incorporated. Add the lemon juice; stir to combine. Add the pork chops back to the pan. Simmer over medium-low heat until sauce thickens slightly, 3 to 4 minutes, basting the chops occasionally with the sauce. Transfer the pork chops to a serving plate.

Drizzle the pork chops with the sauce. Serve chops with the cabbage.

SERVINGS: 4

EGG-FREE
NUT-FREE
SOY-FREE

PREP TIME:
10 MINUTES

COOK TIME:
15 MINUTES

TOTAL TIME:
25 MINUTES

MACROS:

Fat: 72%

Carbs: 5%

Protein: 23%

PER SERVING:

Calories: 645

Total Fat: 50 g

Total Carbs: 8 g

Net Carbs: 6 g

Fiber: 2 g

Sugar: 5 g

Sugar Alcohol: 0 g

Protein: 36 g

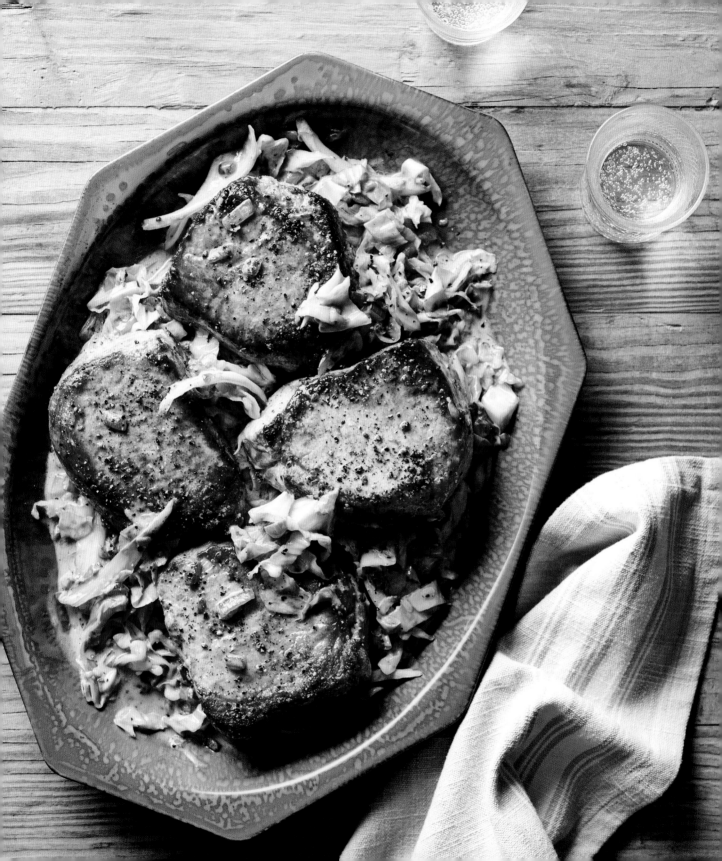

REUBEN CASSEROLE

Deli ingredients that make a tasty, filling, rich, and fast dinner? A way to recreate one of my favorite sandwiches but still keep it keto? Sign me up! The caraway seeds remind me of the rye bread flavor—without the carbs. This casserole makes a lot of liquid once finished. Once it cools a little however, it turns into a thicker sauce that is quite delicious. Drain the sauerkraut well to reduce excess liquid—but don't worry if you get a sauce at the bottom. It's all good.

SERVINGS: 6

NUT-FREE
SOY-FREE

PREP TIME:
10 MINUTES

COOK TIME:
15 MINUTES

TOTAL TIME:
25 MINUTES

COOK TEMPERATURE:
400°F

MACROS:

Fat: 66%

Carbs: 5%

Protein: 29%

PER SERVING:

Calories: 387

Total Fat: 29 g

Total Carbs: 5 g

Net Carbs: 2 g

Fiber: 3 g

Sugar: 1 g

Sugar Alcohol: 0 g

Protein: 29 g

FOR THE RUSSIAN DRESSING

½ cup mayonnaise

2 tablespoons low-sugar ketchup

1 tablespoon minced onion

1 teaspoon hot sauce

1 teaspoon paprika

FOR THE CASSEROLE

1 pound thinly sliced corned beef (or ½ pound each thinly sliced pastrami and corned beef)

2 cups sauerkraut, drained

1 teaspoon caraway seeds

½ pound sliced Swiss cheese

PREHEAT the oven to 400°F.

FOR THE RUSSIAN DRESSING: In a small bowl, stir together the mayonnaise, ketchup, onion, hot sauce, and paprika; set aside.

FOR THE CASSEROLE: Butter a 9- or 8-inch square baking dish. Layer half of the corned beef in the dish. Top with the sauerkraut. Sprinkle with caraway seeds. Drizzle the dressing over the sauerkraut. Top with the remaining corned beef. Top with the cheese.

Bake until the cheese has melted and casserole is bubbling, about 15 minutes. If desired, broil for 2 to 3 minutes to lightly brown the cheese.

SAUSAGE AND BROCCOLI

I hesitate to include simple recipes like this because I don't want people to wonder why they bought a cookbook to get something this simple. But my readers always tell me how much they appreciate these recipes. The main reason I included this is because it's all about the variations. Any type of sausage. Any type of low-carb frozen veggies. Have at it. This recipe, above all others, will be your go-to when you have zero plans for dinner.

SERVINGS: 4

EGG-FREE
NUT-FREE
SOY-FREE

PREP TIME:
5 MINUTES

COOK TIME:
10 MINUTES

TOTAL TIME:
15 MINUTES

MACROS:

Fat: 68%

Carbs: 11%

Protein: 21%

PER SERVING:

Calories: 354

Total Fat: 25 g

Total Carbs: 9 g

Net Carbs: 6 g

Fiber: 3 g

Sugar: 5 g

Sugar Alcohol: 0 g

Protein: 18 g

1 tablespoon extra-virgin olive oil

1 pound smoked sausage, such as kielbasa or chicken sausage, cut into 1-inch pieces

4 cups frozen broccoli (unthawed)

1 cup thinly sliced red bell pepper

1 tablespoon butter

1 teaspoon kosher salt

HEAT A LARGE skillet over medium heat; add the oil. Once the oil is hot, add the sausage. Cook until browned, 2 to 3 minutes. Add the broccoli and ¼ cup water. Cover and cook, stirring once, until broccoli is crisp-tender, 5 to 6 minutes.

Stir in the bell pepper. Add the salt and butter and mix well. Serve hot.

VARIATIONS TO TRY

★ Substitute kale, spinach, green beans, or cauliflower for the broccoli.

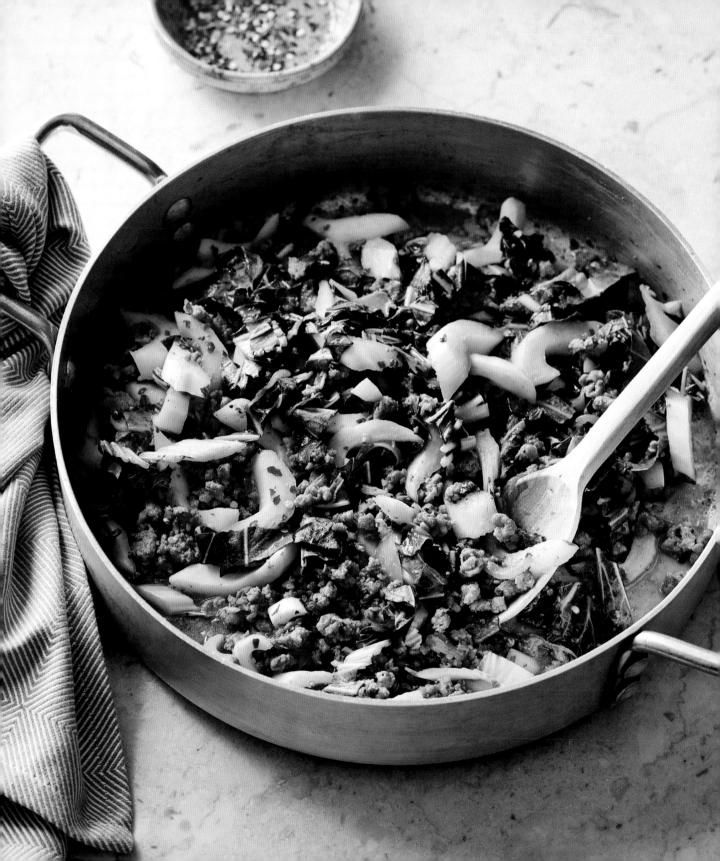

SICHUAN PORK WITH BOK CHOY

You can, of course, use ground beef or chicken if you prefer in this dish. I ask you to add the peanut butter at the end so that you don't have to stand around and guard against it sticking to the bottom of the pan. (Ask me how I know this.) Just be sure it's well-melted and creamy before you serve.

SERVINGS: 4

DAIRY-FREE
EGG-FREE

PREP TIME:
10 MINUTES

COOK TIME:
15 MINUTES

TOTAL TIME:
25 MINUTES

MACROS:

Fat: 71%

Carbs: 8%

Protein: 21%

PER SERVING:

Calories: 455

Total Fat: 36 g

Total Carbs: 9 g

Net Carbs: 7 g

Fiber: 2 g

Sugar: 4 g

Sugar Alcohol: 0 g

Protein: 24 g

2 tablespoons extra-virgin olive oil

1 cup sliced yellow onion

1 pound ground pork

3 cloves garlic, minced

1 teaspoon kosher salt

1 tablespoon Sichuan peppercorns, roughly crushed

1 teaspoon red pepper flakes

1 tablespoon soy sauce

2 packets Splenda

4 cups coarsely chopped bok choy

3 tablespoons peanut butter

HEAT A LARGE skillet over medium heat; add the oil. Once the oil is hot, add the onion and cook until translucent, about 8 minutes.

Add the ground pork and cook, breaking up the meat with a wooden spoon, until cooked through, about 8 minutes.

Push the meat to one side and add the garlic to the pan. Cook just until fragrant, about 30 seconds. Stir in salt, crushed peppercorns, red pepper flakes, soy sauce, sweetener, and ½ cup water.

Bring the mixture to a simmer over medium heat. Stir in the bok choy. Cook until bok choy is crisp-tender, 3 to 5 minutes.

Add the peanut butter and stir until it has melted in to create a sauce.

SKILLET LASAGNA

I do have recipes on the blog where I use zucchini or other vegetables for the "noodles." But the majority of the flavor in a lasagna isn't in the pasta, it's in the fillings. So here, we will just dispense with the pasta and go straight for the fillings. While you could bake this, it comes together rather quickly in a skillet.

SERVINGS: 4

NUT-FREE
SOY-FREE

PREP TIME:
10 MINUTES

COOK TIME:
17 MINUTES

TOTAL TIME:
27 MINUTES

COOK TEMPERATURE:
BROIL

MACROS:

Fat: 63%

Carbs: 5%

Protein: 32%

PER SERVING:

Calories: 520

Total Fat: 36 g

Total Carbs: 7 g

Net Carbs: 7 g

Fiber: 0 g

Sugar: 1 g

Sugar Alcohol: 0 g

Protein: 41 g

FOR THE MEAT LAYER

1 teaspoon extra-virgin olive oil

1 pound 85 percent lean ground beef

¼ cup diced celery

¼ cup diced red onion

1 clove garlic, minced

½ cup low-sugar marinara sauce

1 teaspoon kosher salt

1 teaspoon black pepper

FOR THE CHEESE LAYER

8 ounces ricotta cheese

1 cup mozzarella cheese, shredded

½ cup Parmesan cheese, grated

2 large eggs, lightly beaten

1 teaspoon dried Italian seasoning

½ teaspoon minced garlic

½ teaspoon garlic powder

½ teaspoon black pepper

FOR THE MEAT LAYER: Heat an ovenproof skillet over medium-high heat; add the oil. Once the oil is hot, add the ground beef, celery, onion, and garlic. Cook, breaking up the meat with a wooden spoon, until no longer pink, 5 to 6 minutes.

Stir in the marinara sauce, salt, and pepper. Reduce heat to low. Simmer, stirring occasionally, while you make the cheese layer.

FOR THE CHEESE LAYER: In a large bowl, stir together the ricotta, half of the mozzarella, the Parmesan, eggs, Italian seasoning, minced garlic, garlic powder, and pepper. Spread the cheese mixture over the top of the meat mixture.

Sprinkle with the remaining mozzarella cheese.

Cover and cook on medium-low heat until the cheese is hot and cooked through, 10 to 15 minutes.

Meanwhile, preheat the broiler. Broil lasagna until top is browned, 2 to 3 minutes.

Let stand 10 minutes before serving.

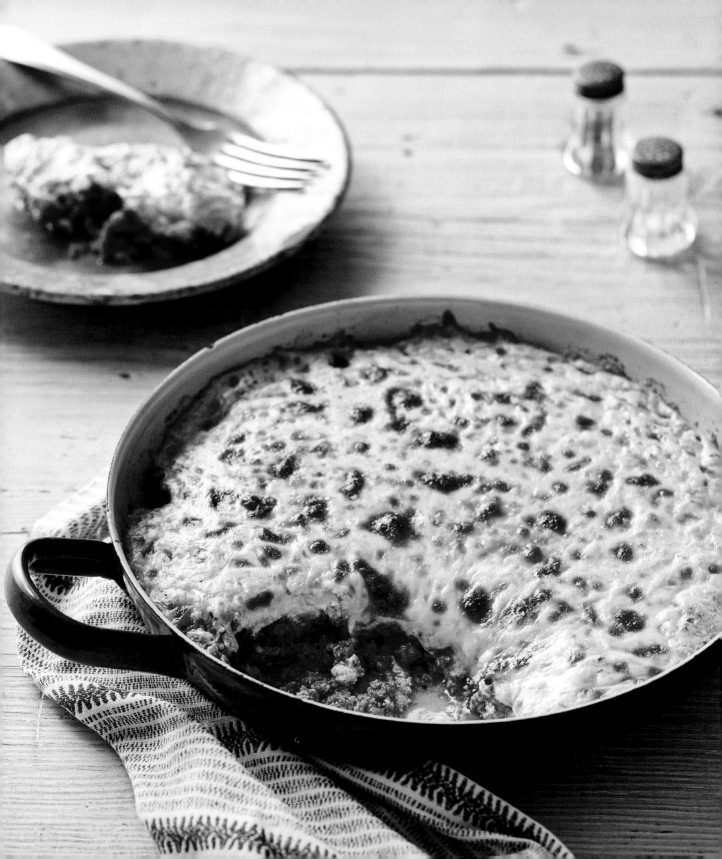

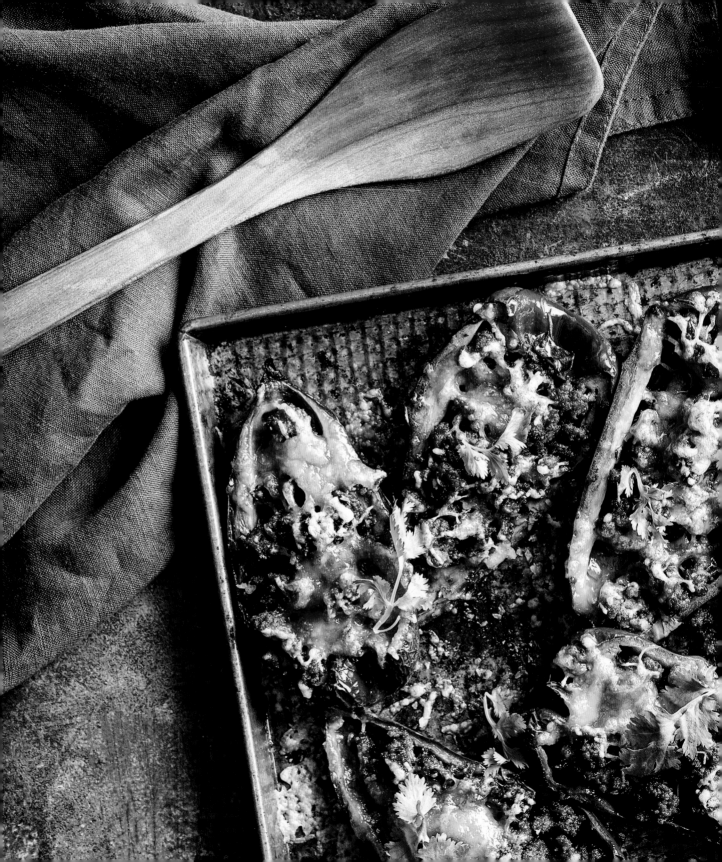

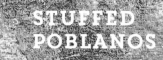

STUFFED
POBLANOS

STUFFED POBLANOS

Roasting the poblanos as you cook the ground beef makes this recipe move ahead lickety-split. Air frying is also an excellent way to roast these peppers. If you have time, you can roast the peppers whole and then stuff them whole. But this way works faster: just laying them flat and layering them with beef and cheese. This feeds four people with the accompaniments or probably two hungry people without the added fat from the sour cream and guacamole.

SERVINGS: 4

EGG-FREE
NUT-FREE
SOY-FREE

PREP TIME:
10 MINUTES

COOK TIME:
6 MINUTES

TOTAL TIME:
16 MINUTES

COOK TEMPERATURE:
BROIL

MACROS:

Fat: 59%

Carbs: 11%

Protein: 30%

PER SERVING:

Calories: 409

Total Fat: 27 g

Total Carbs: 11 g

Net Carbs: 10 g

Fiber: 1 g

Sugar: 1 g

Sugar Alcohol: 0 g

Protein: 30 g

4 large poblano chiles, halved and seeded

1 tablespoon vegetable oil

1 pound 85 percent lean ground beef

1 tablespoon plus 1½ teaspoons taco seasoning

¼ cup chopped fresh cilantro, plus more for garnish

1 cup shredded Mexican blend cheese

Fresh lime juice (optional)

Sour cream (optional)

Guacamole (optional)

PLACE an oven rack 6 inches below the broiler. Preheat the broiler on high.

In a medium bowl, toss the poblano halves with the oil. Arrange, cut side down, on a rimmed sheet pan. Broil until the outsides are charred and blistered, about 4 minutes.

Meanwhile, heat a large skillet over high heat. Add the ground beef and cook, breaking up the meat with a wooden spoon, until cooked through, 6 to 7 minutes. Stir in the taco seasoning and the ¼ cup cilantro.

Fill each poblano half with ground beef and top with cheese. Arrange pepper halves on the baking pan. Broil until the cheese is melted and bubbly, 2 to 3 minutes.

Garnish with additional cilantro, if desired. Serve with a sprinkle of lime juice, sour cream, and/or guacamole, if desired.

EVEN FASTER TIP

You can prepare the poblanos and seasoned meat ahead of time and only assemble one, two, or all four halves, as needed. You'll need to heat the pepper halves and meat in the micro-wave before stuffing the pepper halves, topping with cheese, and broiling.

TEXAS CHILI

I have an Instant Pot version of this chili on the blog as well. What I can tell you is that this chili routinely wins cookoffs at various office events. It's great as leftovers and freezes very well. I freeze it in 1-cup containers, which thaw and heat in a microwave in 3 minutes. Double up and freeze, and you'll always have something in the freezer for the nights you can't cook.

SERVINGS: 4

DAIRY-FREE
EGG-FREE
NUT-FREE
SOY-FREE

PREP TIME:
10 MINUTES

COOK TIME:
10 MINUTES

TOTAL TIME:
20 MINUTES

MACROS:

Fat: 59%

Carbs: 9%

Protein: 32%

PER SERVING:

Calories: 285

Total Fat: 18 g

Total Carbs: 7 g

Net Carbs: 6 g

Fiber: 1 g

Sugar: 3 g

Sugar Alcohol: 0 g

Protein: 22 g

FOR THE CHILI

1 tablespoon extra-virgin oil

½ cup chopped onion

3 cloves garlic, minced

1 pound 85 percent lean ground beef

1 cup canned fire-roasted diced tomatoes

1 tablespoon canned chipotle chiles in adobo sauce, finely chopped

FOR THE SPICE MIX

1 tablespoon Mexican red chile powder

2 teaspoons ground cumin

2 teaspoons kosher salt

1 teaspoon dried oregano

FOR THE CHILI: Heat a large saucepan on medium-high; add the oil. Once the oil is hot, add the onion and garlic. Cook and stir for 30 seconds. Add the ground beef and cook, breaking up the meat with a wooden spoon, until no longer pink, 5 to 6 minutes.

FOR THE SPICE MIX: Meanwhile, in a small bowl, whisk together the chile powder, cumin, salt, and oregano. When the beef is almost cooked through, sprinkle the spice mixture over the meat. Allow the spices to bloom for 30 seconds (do not stir).

Stir in the tomatoes, chipotle chiles, and ½ cup water. Simmer until the tomatoes break down, 4 to 5 minutes.

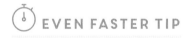 EVEN FASTER TIP

Make up the chili seasoning mix ahead of time.

UNSTUFFED DOLMAS

You won't miss the rice—and you certainly won't miss the time spent rolling dolmas—in this unstuffed dolma dish. It's really so easy, and yet you get all the flavor of dolmas coming through. Don't skip the lemon juice at the end. That little burst of tangy goodness just makes this dish. This casserole freezes very well and tastes even better the next day.

SERVINGS: 4

DAIRY-FREE
EGG-FREE
SOY-FREE

PREP TIME:
10 MINUTES

COOK TIME:
8 MINUTES

TOTAL TIME:
18 MINUTES

MACROS:

Fat: 66%

Carbs: 12%

Protein: 22%

PER SERVING:

Calories: 457

Total Fat: 34 g

Total Carbs: 14 g

Net Carbs: 7 g

Fiber: 7 g

Sugar: 2 g

Sugar Alcohol: 0 g

Protein: 27 g

2 tablespoons extra-virgin olive oil

3 cloves garlic, minced

½ cup chopped onion

1 pound 85 percent lean ground beef or lamb

½ cup pine nuts

1 tablespoon dried parsley or ¼ cup chopped fresh parsley

1 teaspoon ground allspice

1 teaspoon kosher salt

1 teaspoon black pepper

8 ounces brined grape leaves, drained and chopped

3 tablespoons fresh lemon juice

¼ cup chopped fresh mint

HEAT A LARGE skillet on medium-high heat; add the oil. Once the oil is hot, add the garlic and onion. Cook and stir for about 1 minute.

Add the ground beef and pine nuts and cook, breaking up the meat with a wooden spoon, until meat is almost cooked through, 4 to 5 minutes.

Stir in the parsley, allspice, salt, pepper and grape leaves. Cook until the meat has cooked through, 3 to 4 minutes.

Stir in the lemon juice and mint.

INDIVIDUAL MEATLOAVES

Many of us like meatloaf but won't admit this widely. I have no shame about loving meatloaf at all—I just can't use breadcrumbs in mine. I also can't make a sugar-laden glaze for the top, and we all know that meatloaf without a glaze doesn't quite make the grade! In this recipe I ask you to use a little tomato paste for both the glaze and the meatloaf. Not only does this taste good, but it keeps you from wasting most of a can of perfectly good tomato paste. You can double this recipe as easily as you can halve it.

SERVINGS: 4

NUT-FREE
SOY-FREE

PREP TIME:
10 MINUTES

COOK TIME:
24 MINUTES

TOTAL TIME:
34 MINUTES

COOK TEMPERATURE:
350°F/BROIL

MACROS:

Fat: 59%

Carbs: 9%

Protein: 32%

PER SERVING:

Calories: 320

Total Fat: 21 g

Total Carbs: 7 g

Net Carbs: 6 g

Fiber: 1 g

Sugar: 3 g

Sugar Alcohol: 0 g

Protein: 25 g

FOR THE MEATLOAF
1 pound 85 percent lean ground beef

1 large egg

¼ cup almond flour

¼ cup half-and-half

2 tablespoons tomato paste

2 tablespoons Worcestershire sauce

1 teaspoon onion powder

1 teaspoon garlic powder

½ teaspoon kosher salt

1 teaspoon black pepper

FOR THE GLAZE
1 teaspoon yellow mustard

1½ teaspoons tomato paste

1½ teaspoons stevia

PREHEAT the oven to 350°F.

For the meatloaf: In a large bowl, gently mix together the ground beef, egg, almond flour, half-and-half, tomato paste, Worcestershire sauce, onion powder, garlic powder, salt, and pepper. (Keep the mixture loose—don't overwork it or your meatloaf will be tough.)

Divide the mixture into four portions; shape into individual meatloaves. Place a grill rack on a sheet pan or in a square baking dish. Place the meatloaves on the rack. (If you don't have a grill rack that will fit into your baking pan, don't worry about it; just place the meatloaves directly in the pan.) Bake for 20 minutes.

FOR THE GLAZE: Meanwhile, in a small bowl, stir together 2 tablespoons of hot water, mustard, tomato paste, and sweetener and set aside.

Remove the meatloaves from the oven and turn on the broiler. Move the oven rack about 6 inches away from the broiling element.

Brush the tops of the meatloaves with the glaze. Broil until the glaze has browned a little, 4 to 5 minutes. Use a meat thermometer to ensure the meatloaves have reached an internal temperature of 160°F (medium).

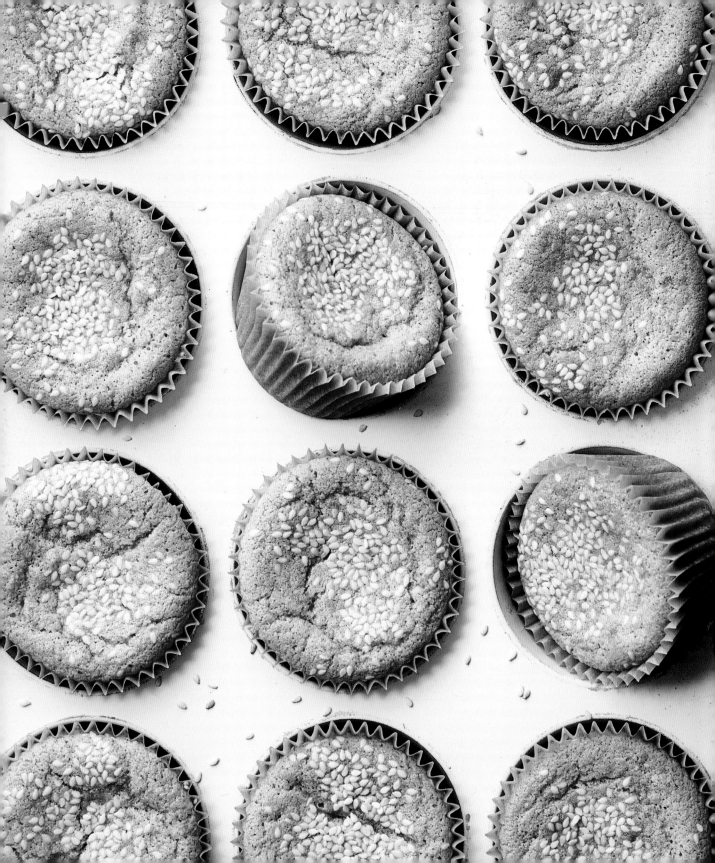

DESSERTS & DRINKS

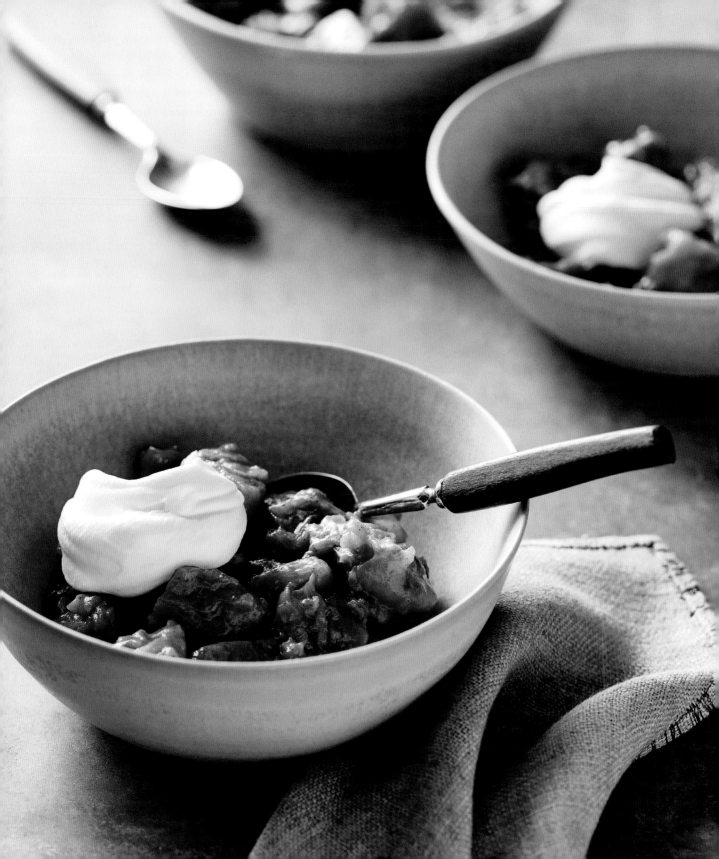

"APPLE PIE" COMPOTE

Except, it's not apples, it's eggplant. Several people in my Twosleevers Keto Facebook group tested this recipe before I posted it because I wanted to make sure it tasted right. I'm so grateful all of them for their help! And you should be too, because although it sounds a little odd, they assure me it tastes just fine. Do not treat the whipped cream as optional in this recipe, as it really helps to offset any remaining eggplant taste.

SERVINGS: 4

EGG-FREE
NUT-FREE
SOY-FREE
VEGETARIAN

PREP TIME:
10 MINUTES

COOK TIME:
10 MINUTES

TOTAL TIME:
16 MINUTES

MACROS:

Fat: 85%

Carbs: 12%

Protein: 3%

PER SERVING:

Calories: 200

Total Fat: 20 g

Total Carbs: 6 g

Net Carbs: 3 g

Fiber: 3 g

Sugar: 4 g

Sugar Alcohol: 0 g

Protein: 2 g

3 tablespoons butter

4 cups chopped and peeled eggplant

¼ cup stevia

2 teaspoons apple pie spice

½ teaspoon xanthan gum

½ cup heavy whipping cream, whipped

HEAT A LARGE skillet over medium-high heat. Add the butter. When the butter is hot, add the eggplant, sweetener, and ½ cup of water. Cook, stirring occasionally, until the eggplant is cooked through, about 5 minutes. Be sure to cook that eggplant down, and don't leave it chewy and chunky. This is key to making it taste like apple pie.

Stir in the apple pie spice and xanthan gum. (If necessary, add an additional ¼ cup or more water.) Cook and stir until the mixture thickens slightly, 1 to 2 minutes.

Serve topped with whipped cream.

5-INGREDIENT ALMOND COOKIES

At Christmas time, I used to make these butter cookies with my sons when they were little—the kind you spritz out of a cookie gun. Over time, the kids grew up, and my rheumatoid arthritis got worse, and I stopped eating flour and sugar. Bye, bye cookies—until I made this recipe. They taste just like those Christmas cookies, except they're a lot faster to make. They also give you two different textures. Soft and moist when warm, and a little crisper when cooled. I enjoy them both ways of course!

Cooking spray
¾ cup Swerve
¼ cup butter, softened
2 large eggs
2 cups almond flour
1 teaspoon almond extract

PREHEAT the oven to 350°F. Spray a large sheet pan with cooking spray; set aside.

In the bowl of a stand mixer fitted with the paddle attachment, combine the sweetener and butter and beat until smooth. Add the eggs and beat until combined. Add the flour and almond extract. Mix until the ingredients are well combined.

Drop by heaping tablespoons onto the prepared sheet pan in 20 portions. Flatten each slightly. Bake until the bottoms are browned and the edges are crispy, 15 to 18 minutes.

Cool on the pan on a wire rack for 5 minutes, then remove from the pan and cool completely on the rack. Store in an airtight container.

VARIATIONS TO TRY

★ Omit the almond extract and add ½ teaspoon ground cinnamon.

★ Substitute lemon extract for the almond extract and add 1 teaspoon lemon zest.

★ Substitute the almond extract for the seeds from a vanilla bean.

SERVINGS: 10 (2 COOKIES EACH)

SOY-FREE VEGETARIAN

PREP TIME: 10 MINUTES

COOK TIME: 15 MINUTES

STAND TIME: 5 MINUTES

TOTAL TIME: 30 MINUTES

COOK TEMPERATURE: 350°F

MACROS:

Fat: 59%

Carbs: 30%

Protein: 10%

PER SERVING:

Calories: 186

Total Fat: 17 g

Total Carbs: 19 g

Net Carbs: 3 g

Fiber: 2 g

Sugar: 1 g

Sugar Alcohol: 14 g

Protein: 6 g

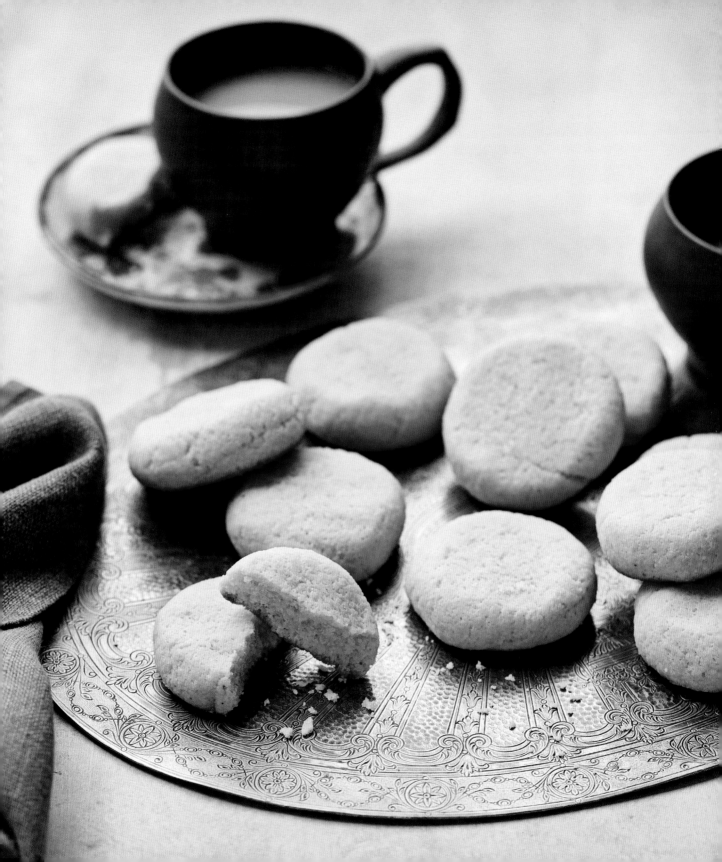

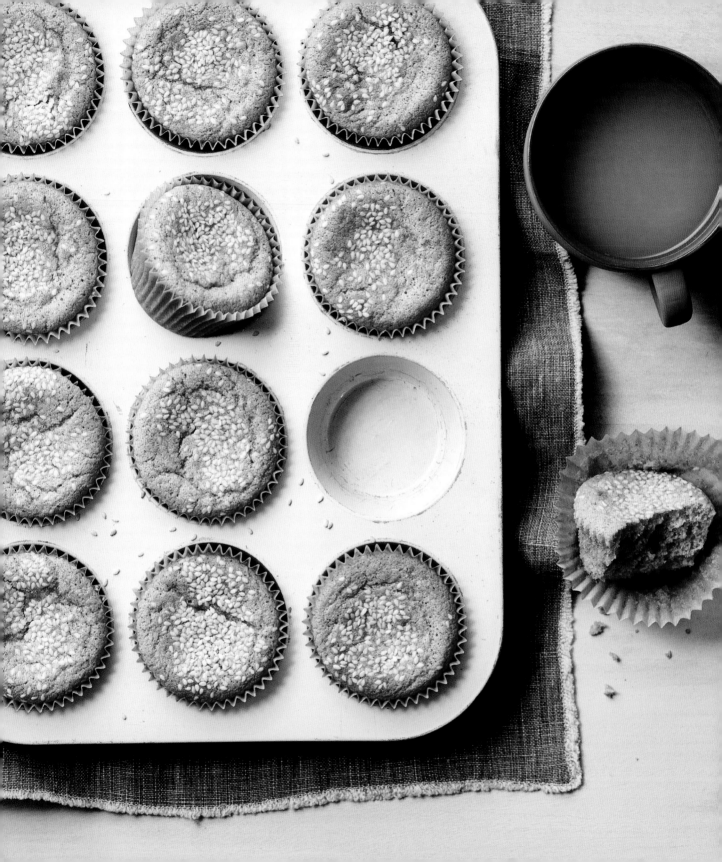

CARDAMOM CUPCAKES

Use this as a base cupcake recipe and change it up with apple pie spice, pumpkin pie spice, or nutmeg. But do try it first with freshly ground cardamom. Sweet, nutty, and warming, this spice will add a little something different to your cakes.

SERVINGS: 12

**SOY-FREE
VEGETARIAN**

PREP TIME:
10 MINUTES

COOK TIME:
25 MINUTES

TOTAL TIME:
35 MINUTES

COOK TEMPERATURE:
350°F

2 cups almond flour

¼ cup unsweetened coconut flakes

1 (13.5-ounce) can coconut milk

½ cup Swerve

¼ cup butter, melted

3 large eggs, beaten

2 teaspoons baking powder

1 teaspoon ground cardamom

¼ cup sesame seeds

PREHEAT the oven to 350°F. Line a 12-cup muffin pan with paper cupcake liners.

In a large skillet pan, toast the almond flour and coconut flakes over medium-high heat, stirring frequently, until and golden brown and lightly toasted, about 5 minutes. Remove from heat. Stir in the coconut milk and allow to stand to absorb the liquid, about 5 minutes.

Transfer the mixture to a large bowl and add the sweetener, butter, eggs, baking powder, and cardamom. Beat with an electric mixer on medium until fluffy.

Divide the batter evenly among the prepared muffin cups. Sprinkle with the sesame seeds.

Bake for 20 minutes, or until a toothpick inserted into the center of one of the cupcakes comes out clean.

Remove the cupcakes from the pan and cool completely on a wire rack.

MACROS:

Fat: 70%

Carbs: 20%

Protein: 10%

PER SERVING:

Calories: 230

Total Fat: 21 g

Total Carbs: 14 g

Net Carbs: 3 g

Fiber: 3 g

Sugar: 2 g

Sugar Alcohol: 8 g

Protein: 7 g

CINNAMON PIE CRUST

Anytime I don't have to roll out pie crust, I consider that a win. I so rarely work with flour anymore that I've entirely lost my touch with rolling out dough, so this pie crust where I just mix and pat out is fast and easy. It tastes particularly good with chocolate fillings.

Cooking spray
1 cup almond flour
2 tablespoons Swerve
1 teaspoon ground cinnamon
¼ cup coconut oil, melted

PREHEAT the oven to 400°F. Spray a 9-inch shallow pie pan with cooking spray; set aside.

In a medium bowl, whisk together the almond flour, sweetener, and cinnamon.

Pour in the coconut oil. Mix until the mixture is crumbly.

Transfer the mixture to the prepared pan. Pat the pie crust evenly into the bottom and up the sides of the pan. Prick the bottom of the crust with a fork.

Bake until firm and golden-brown, about 8 minutes. (If you find the edges starting to brown faster than the rest, either cover the edges with foil, or reduce the temperature to 375°F.)

Cool the crust completely on a wire rack before filling.

> **NOTE**
> ★ The "Apple Pie" Compote (page 209) would be perfect for this crust.

SERVINGS: 8

DAIRY-FREE
EGG-FREE
SOY-FREE
VEGAN

PREP TIME:
5 MINUTES

COOK TIME:
8 MINUTES

COOLING TIME:
20 MINUTES

TOTAL TIME:
33 MINUTES

COOK TEMPERATURE:
400°F

MACROS:

Fat: 77%

Carbs: 16%

Protein: 7%

PER SERVING:

Calories: 141

Total Fat: 14 g

Total Carbs: 6 g

Net Carbs: 1 g

Fiber: 2 g

Sugar: 1 g

Sugar Alcohol: 3 g

Protein: 3 g

ICED CARAMEL MACCHIATO

Make the flavored creamer ahead of time, and your morning bulletproof coffee will be that much faster—and that much tastier. You can, of course, use flavors other than caramel.

SERVINGS: 4

EGG-FREE
SOY-FREE
VEGETARIAN

PREP TIME:
5 MINUTES

COOK TIME:
4 MINUTES

TOTAL TIME:
9 MINUTES

MACROS:

Fat: 95%

Carbs: 2%

Protein: 3%

PER SERVING:

Calories: 263

Total Fat: 28 g

Total Carbs: 1 g

Net Carbs: 1 g

Fiber: 0 g

Sugar: 1 g

Sugar Alcohol: 0 g

Protein: 2 g

¼ cup butter

¼ cup heavy whipping cream

½ cup sugar-free Torani caramel syrup

Ice

2 cups espresso or strong brewed coffee

1 cup plain almond milk

½ cup heavy whipping cream, whipped

COMBINE THE BUTTER and cream in a small saucepan over medium heat. Bring to a boil, stirring frequently. Continue stirring until mixture turns a pale-yellow color and thickens, 4 to 5 minutes.

Slowly add the caramel syrup, stirring constantly. Remove from heat and allow the mixture to cool slightly.

Fill four glasses with ice. Into each glass, pour in ¼ cup almond milk and 2 tablespoons of the caramel sauce; stir.

Pour in the espresso. Do not stir. Top with whipped cream and drizzle with additional caramel sauce, if desired.

COCONUT CHOCOLATE BARK

I've been making this recipe for more than six years now, and it never gets old. I keep it fresh by mixing up what gets added to the chocolate. Coconut, sliced almonds, chopped mixed nuts—all are fair game when I'm on the hunt to make something quick and delicious.

2 tablespoons coconut oil

½ cup unsweetened shredded coconut ¼ cup Swerve

½ cup sugar-free chocolate chips

LINE A SHEET pan with parchment paper; set aside.

Heat a large skillet over medium heat; add the oil. Once the oil is melted, add the coconut and cook, stirring frequently, until lightly browned and toasted, about 5 minutes.

Stir in the sweetener. Remove from the heat and add the chocolate chips. Stir to combine, then allow chocolate to melt.

Spread the mixture onto the parchment paper. Place in the freezer to harden for 10 minutes. (Afterward, it can be stored in the refrigerator.)

Cut into 4 equal pieces.

VARIATIONS TO TRY

★ Use ¼ cup sliced almonds and ¼ cup shredded coconut and toast together.

★ Add 2 tablespoons roasted and salted pepita seeds along with the chocolate.

★ Spoon the candy into little haystacks rather than into a single large pie shape.

SERVINGS: 4

**EGG-FREE
NUT-FREE
SOY-FREE
VEGETARIAN**

PREP TIME:
10 MINUTES

COOK TIME:
5 MINUTES

FREEZING TIME:
10 MINUTES

TOTAL TIME:
25 MINUTES

MACROS:

Fat: 57%

Carbs: 41%

Protein: 2%

PER SERVING:

Calories: 236

Total Fat: 19 g

Total Carbs: 32 g

Net Carbs: 0 g

Fiber: 3 g

Sugar: 1 g

Sugar Alcohol: 29 g

Protein: 1 g

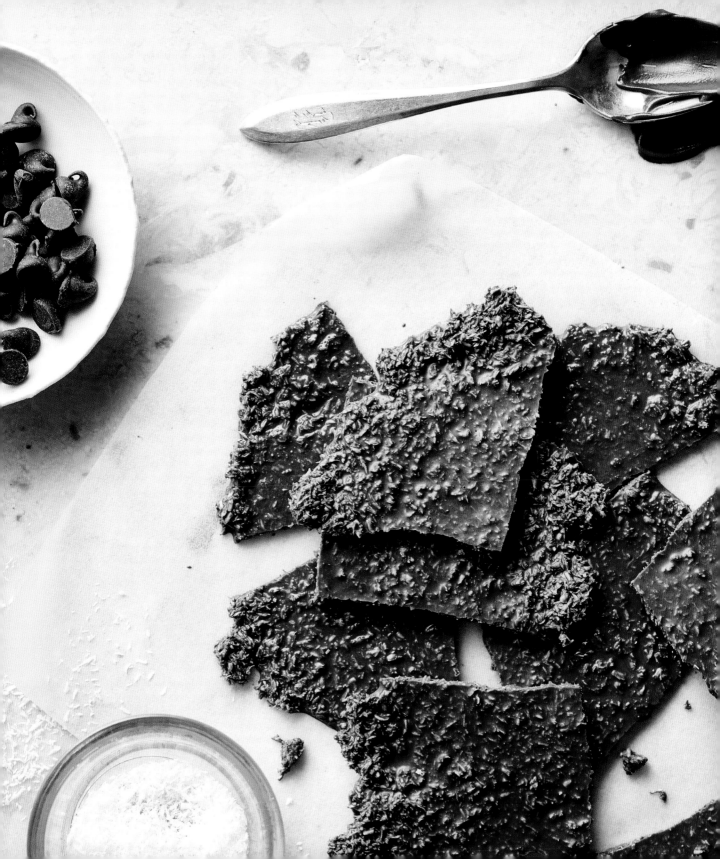

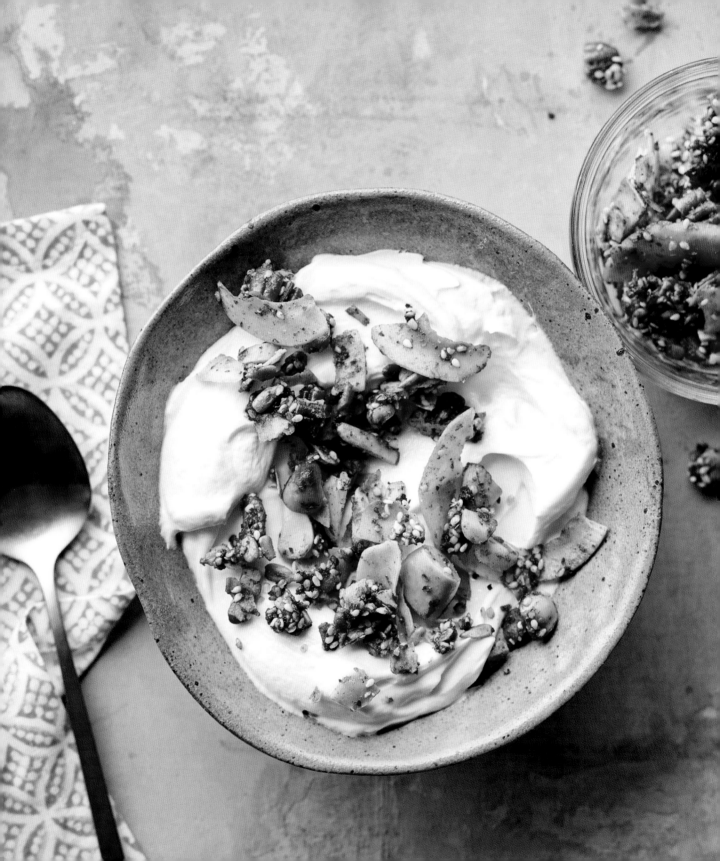

GRANOLA

This won't taste exactly like granola. But it will taste fabulous and it's just perfect with a little milk or almond milk when you're craving crunchy cereal. It's pretty caloric and filling, so start with the recommended ¼ cup per serving and see how far that takes you. Use unsalted nuts and seeds but feel free to use whatever you have at hand. Pecans, macadamia nuts, and Brazil nuts are the lowest in carbs.

SERVINGS: 12
(¼ CUP EACH)

DAIRY-FREE
EGG-FREE
SOY-FREE
VEGAN

PREP TIME:
10 MINUTES

COOK TIME:
5 MINUTES

COOLING TIME:
10 MINUTES

TOTAL TIME:
25 MINUTES

MACROS:

Fat: 75%

Carbs: 17%

Protein: 8%

PER SERVING:

Calories: 201

Total Fat: 20 g

Total Carbs: 10 g

Net Carbs: 2 g

Fiber: 3 g

Sugar: 1 g

Sugar Alcohol: 5 g

Protein: 4 g

3 tablespoons coconut oil or butter

⅓ cup Swerve

2 teaspoons ground cinnamon

½ teaspoon kosher salt

1 cup unsweetened coconut flakes

2 cups mixed nuts and seeds, such as:

½ cup chopped pecans

¼ cup chopped macadamia nuts

¼ cup slivered almonds

¼ cup chopped Brazil nuts

¼ cup sunflower seeds

¼ cup flaxseed meal

¼ cup sesame seeds

¼ cup hemp hearts

Unsweetened almond milk, or full-fat, plain, unsweetened Greek yogurt (optional)

HEAT A SKILLET over medium heat; add the coconut oil. Add the sweetener and cinnamon; stir until incorporated.

Turn the heat to medium-low. Add the coconut flakes, nuts, and seeds; stir to coat. Cook, stirring frequently to keep from burning, until the nuts are toasted, 5 to 8 minutes. Remove from the heat. (The mixture will continue to cook with the residual heat.)

Transfer the mixture to a sheet pan in a single layer to cool and crisp up.

Serve with unsweetened almond milk or Greek yogurt, if desired.

LEMON POUND CAKE

This pound cake is crazy-popular on the blog. People are always commenting about how they snuck this into their non-keto friends, and how everyone raved about it, without realizing it was keto or gluten-free. It makes a fairly large cake as keto cakes go, so it's best to make it for company. This recipe does take a few more than the 30 minutes I promised you, but you can either spend the extra few minutes, or you can make it into cupcakes that bake within 20 minutes.

SERVINGS: 6

**SOY-FREE
VEGETARIAN**

PREP TIME:
10 MINUTES

COOK TIME:
40 MINUTES

COOL TIME:
40 MINUTES

TOTAL TIME:
60 MINUTES

COOK TEMPERATURE:
350°F

MACROS:

Fat: 63%

Carbs: 26%

Protein: 10%

PER SERVING:

Calories: 420

Total Fat: 38 g

Total Carbs: 34 g

Net Carbs: 6 g

Fiber: 4 g

Sugar: 3 g

Sugar Alcohol: 24 g

Protein: 14 g

Cooking spray

¾ cup Swerve

4 tablespoons butter, softened

4 ounces cream cheese, softened

1½ teaspoons lemon extract

Zest of 1 lemon

Juice of 1 lemon

4 large eggs

¼ cup sour cream

2 cups almond flour

2 teaspoons baking powder

PREHEAT the oven to 350°F. Spray a 6-cup Bundt pan or large loaf pan with cooking spray; set aside.

In the bowl of a stand mixer fitted with the paddle attachment, combine the sweetener, butter, and cream cheese. Beat until the mixture is light and fluffy and ingredients are well blended.

Add the lemon extract, lemon zest, and lemon juice; beat to combine. Add the eggs and sour cream and beat until combined. Add the almond flour and baking powder and beat until ingredients are well-blended and the batter is light and fluffy.

Pour the batter into the prepared pan. Bake for 30 to 40 minutes, or until a toothpick inserted into the center of the cake comes out clean.

Cool in the pan on a wire rack for 10 minutes. Remove from the pan and cool completely on a wire rack.

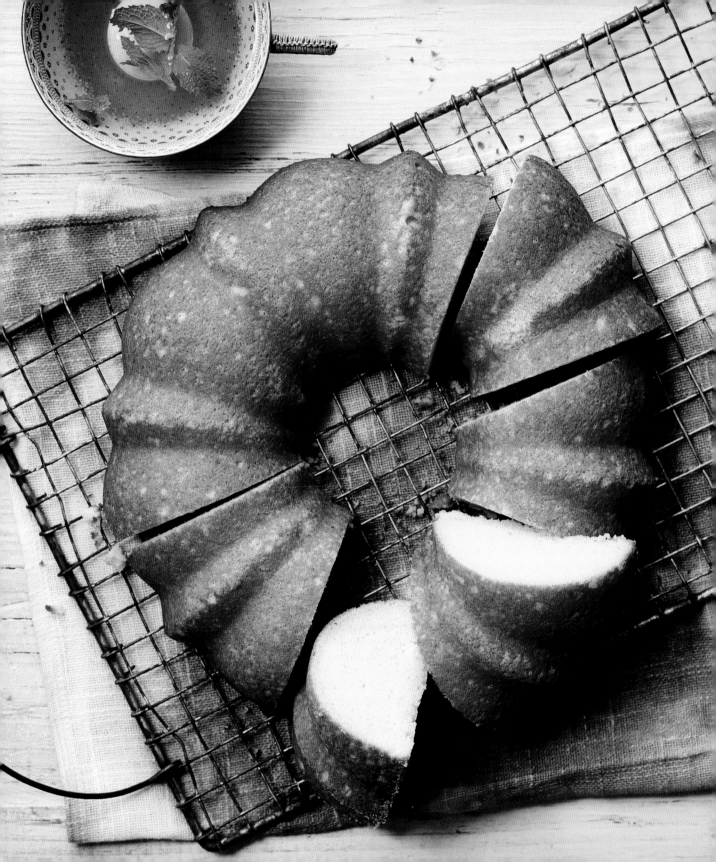

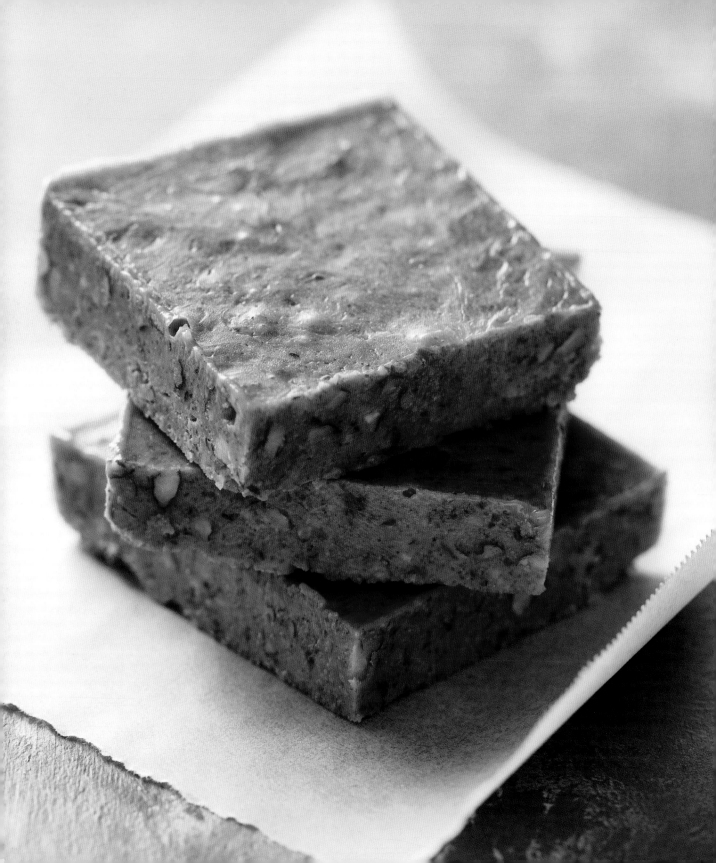

PEANUT PECAN BARS

Here you go. Two minutes to cook a little dessert that makes lovely little snacks for the next few days, using stuff you have in the house. You're welcome! If you're allergic to nuts, use sunflower seed butter and a mix of different seeds such as pumpkin seed, hemp seed, etc. for the topping. Other than that? Melt, mix, pour, freeze, eat.

¾ cup creamy peanut butter

¼ cup coconut oil

¼ cup Swerve

1 teaspoon pure vanilla extract or maple extract

1 cup finely chopped pecans

LINE AN 8-INCH square baking pan with parchment paper.

In a medium microwave-safe bowl, combine the peanut butter, oil, and sweetener. Microwave for 2 minutes, stirring halfway through the cooking time. Stir until ingredients are well-blended.

Add the extract and pecans; stir well. Pour the mixture into the prepared pan.

Freeze until set, about 20 minutes. Cut into 16 squares.

Store in a tightly sealed container for up to 1 week in the refrigerator.

SERVINGS: 16

DAIRY-FREE
EGG-FREE
SOY-FREE
VEGETARIAN

PREP TIME:
5 MINUTES

COOK TIME:
2 MINUTES

FREEZING TIME:
20 MINUTES

TOTAL TIME:
27 MINUTES

MACROS:

Fat: 75%

Carbs: 15%

Protein: 10%

PER SERVING:

Calories: 270

Total Fat: 25 g

Total Carbs: 11 g

Net Carbs: 6 g

Fiber: 2 g

Sugar: 4 g

Sugar Alcohol: 3 g

Protein: 8 g

PEPINO CON LIMON

I love aguas frescas, those delicious, refreshing, fruity flavored drinks of summer. However, they are usually chock-full of sugar, so I have to pass. This Pepino con Limon is fast and refreshing, and of course sugar-free. You can either peel the cucumber for a lighter drink, or leave the peel on for a rich deep green drink. You can either strain it, or drink with the blended-up cucumber in it. Sometimes I throw in a small slice of cantaloupe or honeydew in it, for a little change of pace. I also sometimes add a little hint of chili powder for a surprising tang to it. If you're feeling fancy, reserve a few slices of cucumber to float on top of the drink, and serve with a jaunty little slice of lime waving to you from the rim of the glass.

SERVINGS: 4

DAIRY-FREE
EGG-FREE
NUT-FREE
SOY-FREE
VEGAN

PREP TIME:
10 MINUTES

TOTAL TIME:
10 MINUTES

MACROS:

Fat: 1%

Carbs: 97%

Protein: 2%

PER SERVING:

Calories: 19

Total Fat: 0 g

Total Carbs: 29 g

Ne Carbs: 5 g

Fiber: 0 g

Sugar: 2 g

Sugar Alcohol: 24 g

Protein: 1 g

1 large cucumber, cut into large pieces (peeling optional)

½ cup Truvía

½ cup fresh lime juice

1 cup ice

IN A BLENDER, combine the cucumber, sweetener, lime juice, 2 cups cold water, and ice. Blend until smooth. Strain, if desired. Serve chilled.

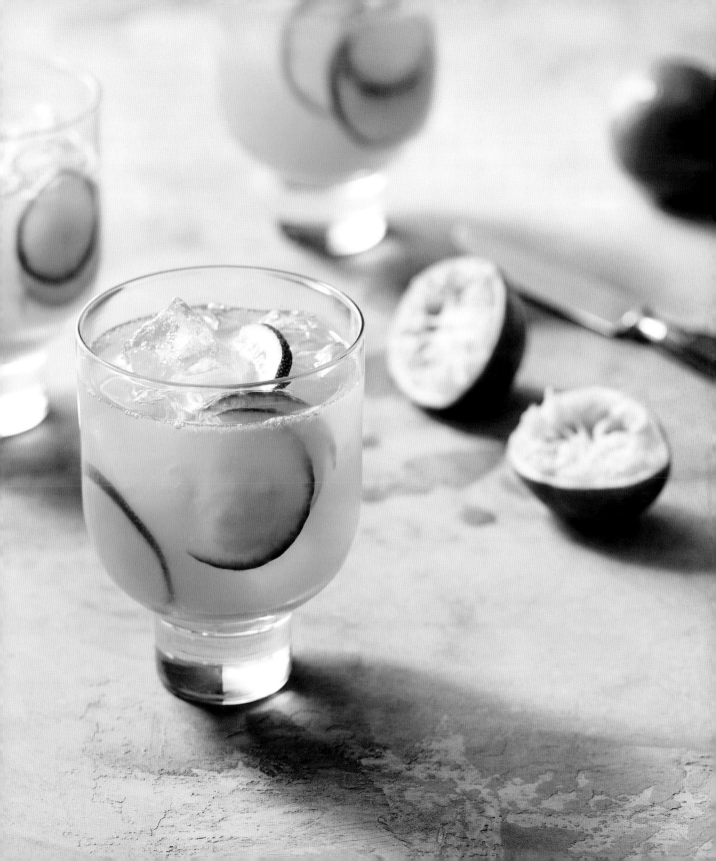

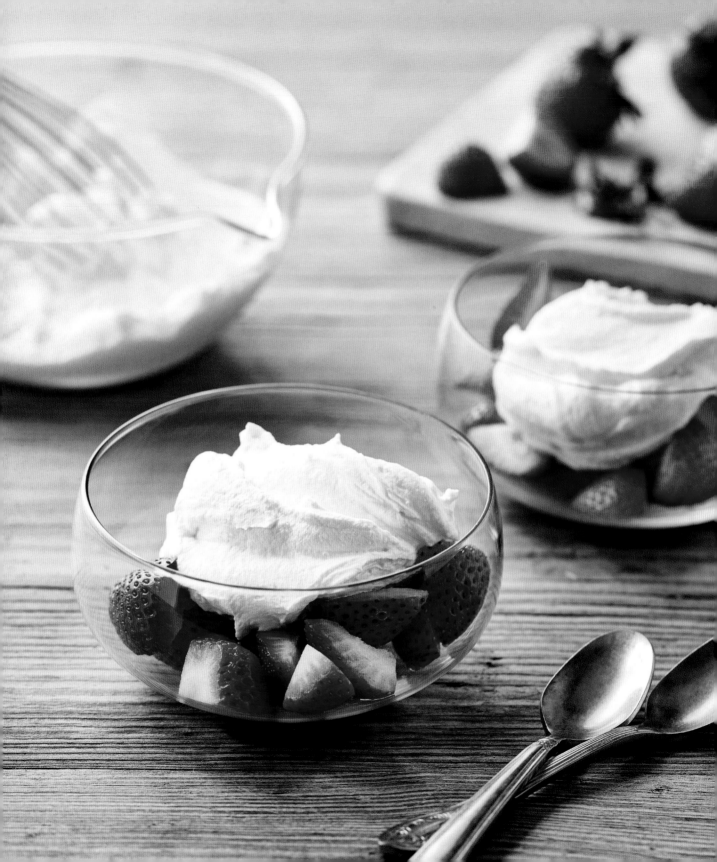

STRAWBERRIES AND CREAM

This makes a lovely, creamy little fat bomb and comes together in minutes. I often used mixed berries in this for a change. If you'd like, you can roughly muddle the berries a bit to get a little more of the berry flavor into the cream. You can also make the Strawberry Jam (page 230) and serve some of that with the cream for a change.

1 cup heavy whipping cream

⅓ cup Truvia

1 teaspoon vanilla or almond extract

8 ounces mascarpone cheese, softened

2 cups chopped fresh strawberries

IN A LARGE BOWL, combine the cream, sweetener, and extract. Beat with an electric mixer until soft peaks form. Add the cheese and whip until the cheese is well incorporated.

Divide the strawberries among 4 cups. Top each cup with one-quarter of the cheese mixture and serve immediately.

SERVINGS: 4

EGG-FREE
NUT-FREE
SOY-FREE
VEGETARIAN

PREP TIME:
10 MINUTES

TOTAL TIME:
10 MINUTES

MARCOS:

Fat: 77%

Carbs: 18%

Protein: 4%

PER SERVING:

Calories: 478

Total Fat: 48 g

Total Carbs: 25 g

Net Carbs: 8 g

Fiber: 1 g

Sugar: 5 g

Sugar Alcohol: 16 g

Protein: 6 g

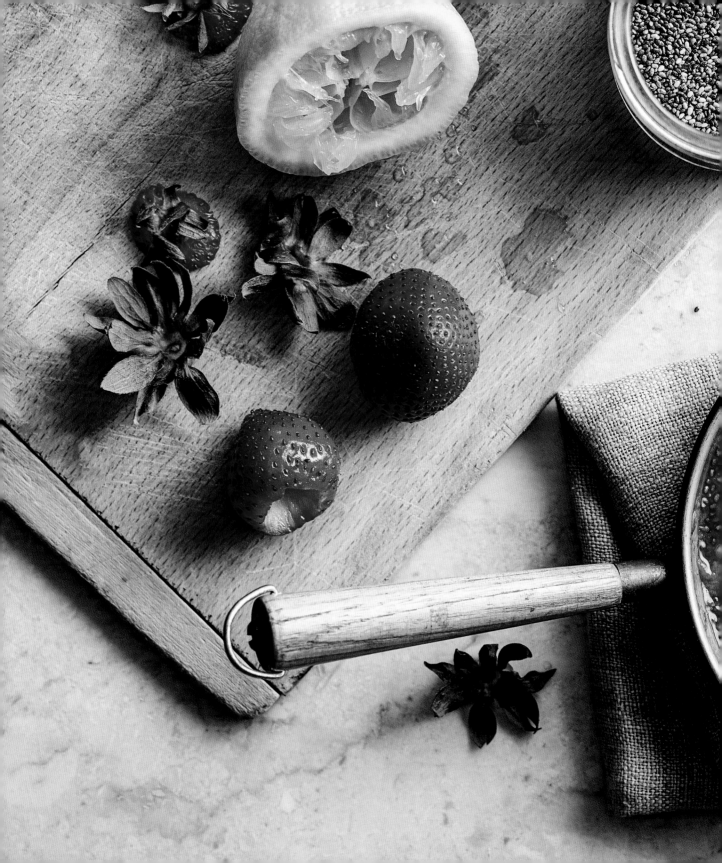

STRAWBERRY JAM

STRAWBERRY JAM

This is a very flexible recipe. You can use any type of berries. You can use this as preserves, as compote, or even as the jelly in the PB&J Shake (page 231). It's fast and it's very handy to have around.

1 cup fresh or frozen strawberries, thawed

1 tablespoon Truvía

1 tablespoon chia seeds

2 teaspoons fresh lemon juice

IN A MEDIUM SAUCEPAN, combine the strawberries, sweetener, and chia seeds with 1 tablespoon of water.

Muddle the strawberries with the back of a spoon to create a rough purée. Cook over medium heat, stirring, until thickened, about 5 minutes.

Remove from the heat and stir in the lemon juice.

Jam may be stored in the refrigerator, covered, for up to 2 weeks.

VARIATIONS TO TRY

★ Substitute any berries of your choice for the strawberries—or use a mix of berries.

★ Add 1 tablespoon of water and use as a compote over desserts.

NOTE

★ Do not use pure erythritol for this recipe as it tends to get grainy when refrigerated.

SERVINGS: 24 (1 TABLESPOON EACH)

DAIRY-FREE
EGG-FREE
NUT-FREE
SOY-FREE
VEGAN

PREP TIME: 5 MINUTES

COOK TIME: 5 MINUTES

TOTAL TIME: 10 MINUTES

MACROS:

Fat: 25%

Carbs: 66%

Protein: 9%

PER SERVING:

Calories: 5

Total Fat: 0 g

Total Carbs: 1 g

Net Carbs: 0 g

Fiber: 0 g

Sugar: 0 g

Sugar Alcohol: 1 g

Protein: 0 g

PB&J SHAKE

Who doesn't love PB&J? I sometimes make this with fresh strawberries, but the carb counts tend to be a little higher with that version. This is a comforting, easy shake for breakfast or for a snack.

2 cups ice

2 cups almond milk

2 tablespoons peanut butter

2 tablespoons Strawberry Jam (page 230)

1 scoop unflavored whey protein (optional)

3 to 4 teaspoons Truvía

IN A BLENDER, combine the ice, almond milk, peanut butter, Strawberry Jam, whey protein (if using), and sweetener. Blend until smooth. Divide between two glasses; serve immediately.

SERVINGS: 2

DAIRY-FREE
EGG-FREE
SOY-FREE
VEGAN

PREP TIME:
5 MINUTES

TOTAL TIME:
5 MINUTES

MACROS:

Fat: 60%

Carbs: 29%

Protein: 11%

PER SERVING:

Calories: 130

Total Fat: 11 g

Total Carbs: 12 g

Net Carbs: 4 g

Fiber: 1 g

Sugar: 2 g

Sugar Alcohol: 7 g

Protein: 5 g

SAUCES, DRESSINGS & SPICE MIXES

ALL-PURPOSE MUSTARD DRESSING

This is a great all-purpose dressing. I often use it as a glaze over meats. When you heat the dressing, it makes a lovely sauce that can be served with grilled meats. Since it keeps for a week in the refrigerator, it's a great savory fat bomb to keep around for flavor.

MAKES:
ABOUT ¾ CUP

DAIRY-FREE
EGG-FREE
NUT-FREE
VEGAN

TOTAL TIME:
5 MINUTES

¼ cup apple cider vinegar

1 teaspoon soy sauce

½ cup extra-virgin olive oil

¼ teaspoon kosher salt

¼ teaspoon black pepper

2 cloves garlic, minced

1 packet Splenda

1 tablespoon Dijon mustard

IN A BLENDER container combine the vinegar, soy sauce, oil, salt, pepper, garlic, sweetener, and mustard. Blend until smooth. Store in a tightly sealed container in the refrigerator for up to 1 week.

ASIAN PEANUT SAUCE

This is perfect to use as a salad dressing, as a satay dipping sauce, or for air-fried tofu. This sauce will keep in the fridge for 1 week.

MAKES:
ABOUT 1 CUP

DAIRY-FREE
EGG-FREE
VEGAN

TOTAL TIME:
5 MINUTES

⅓ cup peanut butter

2 tablespoons soy sauce

2 tablespoons rice wine vinegar

Juice of 1 lime

1 teaspoon minced fresh ginger

1 clove garlic, minced

1 teaspoon black pepper

IN A BLENDER CONTAINER, combine the peanut butter, soy sauce, vinegar, lime juice, ginger, garlic, pepper, and ¼ cup hot water. Blend until smooth.

Use immediately or store in a tightly sealed container in the refrigerator up to 1 week.

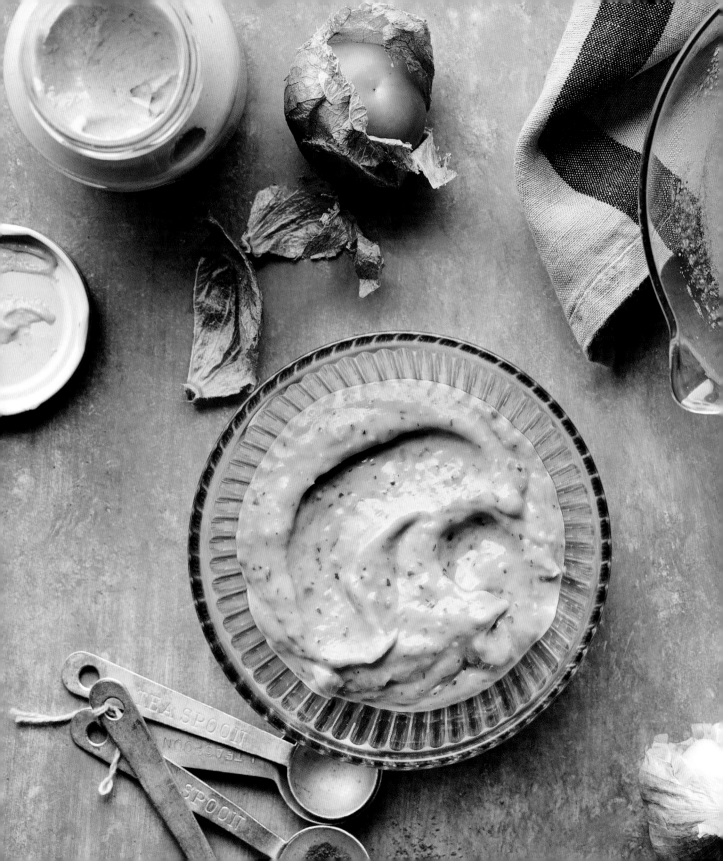

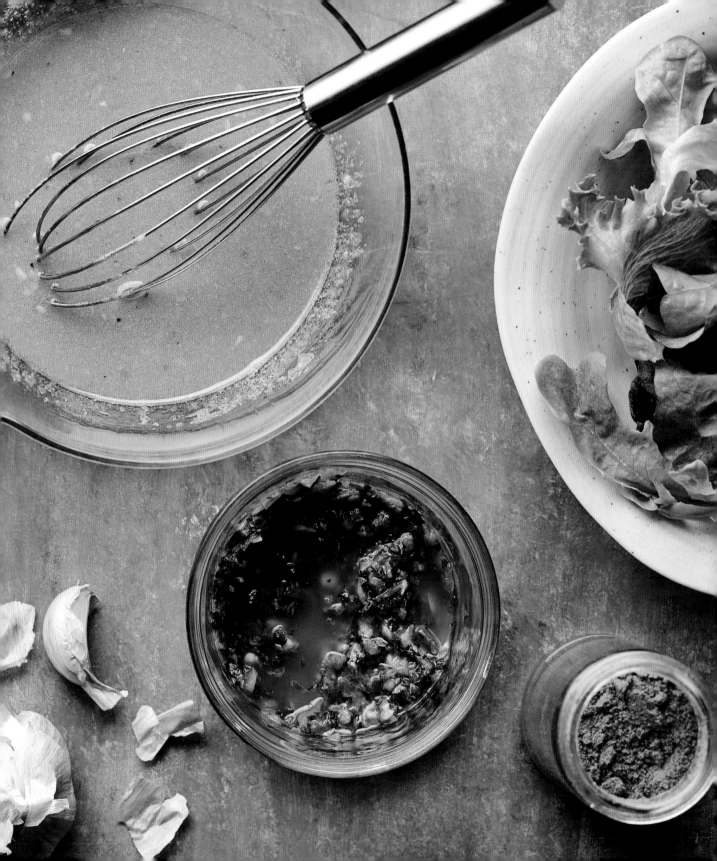

AVOCADO TOMATILLO DRESSING

If you have a better recipe for an easy, spicy, creamy, authentic tomatillo salsa, I need to see it immediately. Because if not, I am going to claim that this is the BEST tomatillo salsa you've ever had. I have no shame about saying this because I got this from Nora in my Facebook group—and we are all addicted to it.

MAKES:
ABOUT 4 CUPS

EGG-FREE
NUT-FREE
SOY-FREE
VEGETARIAN

PREP TIME:
5 MINUTES

COOK TIME:
5 MINUTES

TOTAL TIME:
10 MINUTES

6 medium tomatillos, husked and rinsed

2 serrano chile peppers, stemmed and seeded

¼ cup chopped fresh cilantro

½ teaspoon salt

1 large avocado, halved, pitted, and peeled

1 clove garlic, coarsely chopped

2 tablespoons Mexican crema or full-fat sour cream

IN A LARGE saucepan combine the tomatillos, serrano peppers, and water to cover. Bring to a boil over high heat. Reduce heat and cook until tomatillos are just tender but not mushy, about 5 minutes; drain.

Transfer tomatillos and chiles to a blender. Add the cilantro, salt, avocado, garlic, and crema. Blend until smooth. Taste and adjust salt and crema, if necessary.

CILANTRO-JALAPEÑO DRESSING

Don't be misled by the handful of ingredients in this super-tasty dressing. Fast, addictive, and usable for a variety of purposes, this dressing will be a favorite to keep on hand. My readers tell me all the time how they end up eating this dressing with a spoon.

MAKES: ABOUT ¾ CUP

EGG-FREE
NUT-FREE
SOY-FREE
VEGETARIAN

TOTAL TIME:
5 MINUTES

½ cup full-fat sour cream

½ cup chopped fresh cilantro

½ jalapeño, seeded

¼ teaspoon kosher salt

¼ teaspoon black pepper

6 cloves garlic, minced

IN A BLENDER or food processor, combine the sour cream, cilantro, jalapeño, salt, pepper, and garlic. Blend or process until smooth.

TANGY TAMARIND VINAIGRETTE

The tamarind paste in this recipe really makes this salad sing. You can get this online or in Asian grocery stores. This is a great example of something that can be used as a salad dressing or as a marinade. Use it for the Tangy Shrimp Salad (page 79) or with the salad of your choice.

MAKES: ABOUT ¾ CUP

DAIRY-FREE
EGG-FREE
NUT-FREE

PREP TIME:
5 MINUTES

COOK TIME:
2 MINUTES

COOLING TIME:
20 MINUTES

TOTAL TIME:
27 MINUTES

2 tablespoons soy sauce

2 tablespoons fish sauce

2 tablespoons tamarind paste

2 tablespoons vinegar

2 tablespoons Truvía

1 tablespoon sambal oelek

1 tablespoon fresh lime juice

IN A MEDIUM microwave-safe bowl, stir together 2 tablespoons of water with the soy sauce, fish sauce, tamarind paste, vinegar, sweetener, sambar oelek, and lime juice. Microwave for 2 minutes or until bubbling. (Or heat on the stove, allowing it to boil for 1 to 2 minutes.)

Cool completely, then store in a tightly sealed container in the refrigerator for up to 2 weeks.

ETHIOPIAN NITER KIBBEH

Your house will smell so good when you make this! Niter Kibbeh is clarified butter with aromatics and spices in it. It's easy to make—and even easier to eat and enjoy on vegetables, in stews, and anywhere else where you might use ghee or butter.

MAKES:
1½ CUPS

EGG-FREE
NUT-FREE
SOY-FREE
VEGETARIAN

PREP TIME:
10 MINUTES

COOK TIME:
30 MINUTES

TOTAL TIME:
40 MINUTES

1 pound unsalted butter

4 cloves garlic, minced

1 yellow onion, chopped

1 tablespoon minced fresh ginger

1½ teaspoons black pepper

½ teaspoon ground turmeric

1 teaspoon cardamom seeds

1 teaspoon fenugreek seeds

½ teaspoon cumin seeds

1 to 2 cinnamon sticks

4 whole cloves

IN A MEDIUM SAUCEPAN, combine the butter, garlic, onion, ginger, pepper, turmeric, cardamom seeds, fenugreek seeds, cumin seeds, cinnamon sticks, and cloves. Bring to a simmer over medium heat. Cook until the bubbles rising to the top are clear and the mixture is no longer milky, about 30 minutes.

Place a fine-mesh strainer over a heatproof jar (such as a 2-cup mason jar). Strain the mixture into the jar; discard the solids. Cover and store in the refrigerator or freezer.

VARIATIONS TO TRY

★ If you eat vegan, substitute 14 to 15 ounces of coconut oil for the unsalted butter.

HOMEMADE GHEE

I don't understand why it's so expensive to buy ghee in stores because really, it's fairly idiot-proof to make this at home. Let it boil, turn down the heat until the ghee is at a simmering boil, and 20 minutes later you have ghee, which keeps forever on your countertop in a sealed container. OR at least, as long as it takes for you to devour it—which isn't very long at our house.

MAKES: 2 CUPS

EGG-FREE
NUT-FREE
SOY-FREE
VEGETARIAN

COOK TIME:
25 MINUTES

TOTAL TIME:
25 MINUTES

1 pound unsalted butter

PLACE THE BUTTER in a heavy-bottomed saucepan. Place the pan over medium-low heat. Set a timer for 20 minutes and LEAVE IT ALONE! Don't stir the butter or mess with it in any way. Just let it be. (During this time, the water from the butter will evaporate. You will see a light foam forming on the top of the bubbling butter. It will sound like popcorn popping—but much softer.)

At the 20-minute mark, stir the butter and turn the heat to medium-high. Cook, stirring occasionally, until you see the milk solids start turning brown and settling into the bottom of the pan. If you give up before this stage you are either: (a) a quitter or (b) trying to make clarified butter, not ghee.

Let the mixture cool a little, then strain the clear yellow liquid through a fine-mesh strainer into a jar with a lid. (Discard the brown milk solids.) Seal the jar tightly, and you're done.

You can store the ghee on your countertop for months on end. As long as you keep it sealed and use a clean spoon each time you dig into it, ghee lasts almost indefinitely.

TZATZIKI WITH TAHINI

It seems to me that Mediterranean, Middle Eastern, and Indian cuisines all share some version of dishes that combine cooling yogurt with some kind of vegetable. Whether it's an Indian raita, a Persian *borani*, or a Greek tzatziki, the combination of yogurt, veggies, and a few little spices makes a great sauce to accompany all kinds of grilled meats.

MAKES: ABOUT 3 CUPS

EGG-FREE
NUT-FREE
SOY-FREE
VEGETARIAN

TOTAL TIME:
10 MINUTES

1 large cucumber, peeled and grated (about 2 cups)

1 cup plain full-fat, plain, unsweetened Greek yogurt

2 to 3 cloves garlic, minced

1 tablespoon tahini (sesame paste)

1 tablespoon fresh lemon juice

½ teaspoon salt

Chopped fresh parsley or dill, for garnish (optional)

IN A MEDIUM bowl combine the cucumber, yogurt, garlic, tahini, lemon juice, and salt. Stir until well combined. Cover and chill until ready to serve.

Right before serving, sprinkle with chopped fresh parsley, if desired.

ZHOUG

If you are one of those that can't do cilantro, try this Zhoug with parsley instead. It's a fresh, herby sauce that I use with both vegetables and meats.

MAKES:
ABOUT ¾ CUP

DAIRY-FREE
EGG-FREE
NUT-FREE
SOY-FREE
VEGAN

TOTAL TIME:
10 MINUTES

1 cup packed fresh cilantro

2 cloves garlic, peeled

2 jalapeño or serrano chiles, stemmed and coarsely chopped

½ teaspoon ground cumin

¼ teaspoon ground coriander

¼ teaspoon kosher salt

2 to 4 tablespoons extra-virgin olive oil

IN A FOOD PROCESSOR, combine the cilantro, garlic, jalapeños, cumin, coriander, and salt. Process until finely chopped. Add 2 tablespoons olive oil and pulse to form a loose paste, adding up to 2 tablespoons more olive oil if needed.

Transfer the zhoug to a glass container. Cover and store in the refrigerator until 30 minutes before serving.

CAJUN SPICE

You can certainly use a store-bought Cajun spice mix—but I like making it at home so that I can play with the proportions. I like to add more cayenne than what I have listed here, so you can always use more (or less!) than the 1 teaspoon.

MAKES:
ABOUT ⅓ CUP

DAIRY-FREE
EGG-FREE
NUT-FREE
SOY-FREE
VEGAN

TOTAL TIME:
5 MINUTES

1 teaspoon dried oregano

1 teaspoon dried thyme

1 tablespoon dried parsley flakes

1 tablespoon dehydrated minced onion

1 teaspoon dehydrated minced garlic

1 tablespoon smoked paprika

1 teaspoon cayenne pepper

1 teaspoon black pepper

1 teaspoon kosher salt

IN A SMALL BOWL, stir together the oregano, thyme, parsley flakes, onion, garlic, paprika, cayenne pepper, black pepper, and salt. Store in an airtight container in a cool, dark place for up to 2 months.

HARISSA

Many harissa recipes use tomatoes or peppers. I prefer my paste to be straight-up spice. Taste it once and you will find a million different uses for this lovely, spicy, versatile mix.

½ cup vegetable oil

6 cloves garlic, minced

2 tablespoons smoked paprika

1 tablespoon ground coriander

1 tablespoon ground cumin

1 teaspoon ground caraway

1 teaspoon kosher salt

½ to 1 teaspoon cayenne pepper

IN A MEDIUM microwave-safe bowl, stir together the vegetable oil, garlic, paprika, coriander, cumin, caraway, salt, and cayenne. Microwave on high for 1 minute, stirring halfway through the cooking time. (You can also heat this on the stovetop until the vegetable oil is hot and bubbling.)

Cool completely before storing in an airtight container in the refrigerator for up to 1 month.

MAKES:
ABOUT 1 CUP

DAIRY-FREE
EGG-FREE
NUT-FREE
SOY-FREE
VEGAN

PREP TIME:
5 MINUTES

COOK TIME:
1 MINUTE

COOLING TIME:
20 MINUTES

TOTAL TIME:
26 MINUTES

RAS AL HANOUT

Once again, recipes for this heady mix vary family by family, and shop by shop, since the name simply means "top of the shop," or the best of what the shop has to offer. When I'm feeling extravagant, I add liberal amounts of saffron, but most days I find the recipe below to be just right for us.

2 teaspoons ground cumin

2 teaspoons ground ginger

2 teaspoons ground turmeric

1 teaspoon ground cardamom

1 teaspoon ground cinnamon

w1 teaspoon cayenne pepper

1 teaspoon ground allspice

2 teaspoons kosher salt

2 teaspoons black pepper

IN A SMALL BOWL, stir together the cumin, ginger, turmeric, cardamom, cinnamon, coriander, cayenne pepper, allspice, salt, and black pepper. Store in an airtight container in a cool, dark place for up to 2 months.

MAKES: ⅓ CUP

DAIRY-FREE
EGG-FREE
NUT-FREE
SOY-FREE
VEGAN

TOTAL TIME:
5 MINUTES

INDIAN GARAM MASALA

This garam masala is the base of much of my Indian cooking. I've tried many different recipes, but this is Raghavan Iyer's recipe (he of *660 Curries* fame), and he has been generous enough to allow me and all who cook from my recipes to use this. Everyone who has tried it will agree—store-bought garam masalas cannot hold a candle to this recipe. Take my advice—take the 10 minutes it takes to make this. You will thank me.

MAKES: ¼ CUP

DAIRY-FREE
EGG-FREE
NUT-FREE
SOY-FREE
VEGAN

TOTAL TIME:
10 MINUTES

2 tablespoons coriander seeds

1 teaspoon cumin seeds

½ teaspoon whole black cloves

½ teaspoon cardamom seeds (from green/white pods)

2 dried bay leaves

3 dried red chiles or ½ teaspoon cayenne pepper or red pepper flakes

1 (2-inch) piece cinnamon or cassia bark

COMBINE CORIANDER SEEDS, cumin seeds, cloves, cardamom seeds, bay leaves, chiles, and cinnamon in a clean coffee or spice grinder. Grind, shaking as it's being ground, so all the seeds and bits get into the blades, until mixture has the consistency of a moderately fine powder.

Unplug the grinder and turn it upside down. (You want all the spice mixture to collect in the lid so you can easily scoop it out without cutting yourself playing about the blades.)

Transfer the garam masala to an airtight container and store in a cool, dark place for up to 2 months.

DIETARY CONSIDERATIONS

RECIPE	PAGE	DAIRY FREE	EGG FREE	NUT FREE	SOY FREE	VEGETARIAN	VEGAN	COOK TIME	NET CARBS	TOTAL CARBS
ANTIPASTO SALAD WITH PESTO VINAIGRETTE	59		X		X				1 g	4 g
ASIAN CHICKEN SALAD	60	X	X						4 g	7 g
BIG MAC SALAD	63			X	X			7 minutes	3 g	7 g
CREAMY BROCCOLINI BACON SALAD	64				X				9 g	13 g
CABBAGE COCONUT SLAW	67	X	X		X	X	X	30 seconds	5 g	8 g
CEVICHE AVOCADO	68	X	X	X	X				8 g	18 g
CREAMY CHICKEN SALAD	69	X			X				1 g	2 g
CUCUMBER PEANUT SLAW	70	X	X		X	X	X	30 seconds	3 g	5 g
HEMP HEART TABBOULEH	73	X	X	X	X	X	X		5 g	8 g
SICHUAN SMASHED CUCUMBERS	74	X	X			X	X		6 g	9 g
SPICY KOREAN CUCUMBER SALAD	78	X	X	X	X	X	X		6 g	7 g
TANGY SHRIMP SALAD	79	X		X	X				5 g	8 g
ASPARAGUS MUSHROOM STIR FRY	83	X	X	X				3 minutes	4 g	7 g
CAULIFLOWER BREADSTICKS	84			X	X	X		32 minutes	1 g	2 g
CREAMED SPINACH	86		X	X	X	X		25 minutes	10 g	12 g
ETHIOPIAN COLLARD GREENS (GOMEN WOT)	87	X	X	X	X	X	X	17 minutes	7 g	12 g
HARISSA-ROASTED TURNIPS	89	X	X	X	X	X	X	10 minutes	9 g	13 g
RAJAS CON CREMA	90		X	X	X	X		8 minutes	10 g	11 g
ROASTED RATATOUILLE	93	X	X	X	X	X	X	20 minutes	10 g	15 g

DIETARY CONSIDERATIONS (CONTINUED)

RECIPE	PAGE	DAIRY FREE	EGG FREE	NUT FREE	SOY FREE	VEGETARIAN	VEGAN	COOK TIME	NET CARBS	TOTAL CARBS
SHEET PAN OKRA MASALA	94	X	X	X	X	X	X	15 minutes	9 g	14 g
SPICY CREAM OF MUSHROOM SOUP	96		X	X	X			15 minutes	10 g	13 g
VEGETABLES IN CREAM SAUCE	97			X	X			10 minutes	9 g	12 g
SWISS CHARD WITH GARLIC AND PINE NUTS	99	X	X		X			11 minutes	5 g	6 g
CAULIFLOWER MAC AND CHEESE WITH BACON AND JALAPEÑOS	103		X	X	X			16 minutes	5 g	6 g
CHEESE CRISPS	104		X	X	X	X		90 seconds	0 g	0 g
HOT AND SOUR EGG DROP SOUP	106	X		X				5 minutes	2 g	2 g
BROCCOLI CHEESE SOUP	107		X	X	X			15 minutes	7 g	9 g
PANEER TIKKA	109		X	X	X	X		4 minutes	5 g	6 g
SOUTHWESTERN FRITTATA	110			X	X			12 minutes	4 g	5 g
QUESO FUNDIDO	112		X	X	X			20 minutes	8 g	10 g
ARTICHOKE CHICKEN SOUP	118		X	X	X			20 minutes	8 g	11 g
BUFFALO CHICKEN CASSEROLE	119		X	X	X			15 minutes	3 g	4 g
BROCCOLI CHICKEN BAKE	121		X		X			15 minutes	5 g	9 g
CHICKEN BIRYANI	122	X	X	X	X			20 minutes	4 g	6 g
CHICKEN CORDON BLEU CASSEROLE	124		X	X	X			20 minutes	4 g	4 g
CHICKEN POT PIE SOUP	125		X	X	X			20 minutes	7 g	9 g
CREAMY TUSCAN CHICKEN	127		X	X	X			20 minutes	8 g	10 g
FRENCH GARLIC CHICKEN	128		X	X	X			20 minutes	4 g	4 g

RECIPE	PAGE	DAIRY FREE	EGG FREE	NUT FREE	SOY FREE	VEGETARIAN	VEGAN	COOK TIME	NET CARBS	TOTAL CARBS
PUNJABI DRY CHICKEN CURRY	131	X	X	X	X			15 minutes	3 g	4 g
SOUR CREAM SKILLET CHICKEN ENCHILADAS	132		X	X	X			26 minutes	4 g	5 g
TACOS DE ALAMBRE	135		X	X	X			15 minutes	4 g	5 g
TOM KHA GAI SOUP	138	X	X	X	X			10 minutes	7 g	9 g
SPICED CHICKEN MEATBALLS	139	X	X	X	X			10 minutes	1 g	2 g
BUTTERY SAUSAGE AND SHRIMP	147		X	X	X			5 minutes	3 g	3 g
HOT WING SCALLOPS	148		X	X	X			5 minutes	5 g	5 g
SALMON DIP	149		X		X				2 g	3 g
MISO SALMON CHOWDER	151	X	X	X				10 minutes	7 g	9 g
PESTO SALMON WITH GARLIC SPINACH	152		X		X			15 minutes	10 g	13 g
SHRIMP AND ASPARAGUS GRIBICHE	155	X		X	X			10 minutes	4 g	6 g
SHRIMP AND GRITS	156		X	X	X			10 minutes	7 g	9 g
SHRIMP WITH FETA AND TOMATOES	159		X	X	X			10 minutes	6 g	8 g
SHRIMP WITH TOMATILLOS AND COTIJA	160		X	X	X			16 minutes	10 g	12 g
SMOKED SALMON AND CHEESE TIMBALE	163		X	X	X				3 g	4 g
SPICY TUNA SALAD	164	X	X						7 g	12 g
GREEN CURRY MUSSELS	168	X	X	X				15 minutes	10 g	12 g
SMOKY SHRIMP SCAMPI	169		X	X	X			5 minutes	2 g	2 g
BEEF SHAWARMA	172	X	X	X	X			15 minutes	5 g	8 g
BEEF STROGANOFF	173		X	X	X			15 minutes	7 g	9 g
CAJUN DIRTY RICE	174	X	X	X	X			15 minutes	7 g	10 g

DIETARY CONSIDERATIONS (CONTINUED)

RECIPE	PAGE	DAIRY FREE	EGG FREE	NUT FREE	SOY FREE	VEGETARIAN	VEGAN	COOK TIME	NET CARBS	TOTAL CARBS
EASY TACO DIP	175		X	X	X			15 minutes	7 g	8 g
CHEATER YUKGAEJANG	177	X		X				15 minutes	2 g	3 g
FLANK STEAK FAJITAS	178	X	X	X	X			15 minutes	6 g	8 g
HARISSA LAMB CHOPS AND KALE	181		X	X	X			15 minutes	7 g	11 g
ITALIAN SAUSAGE AND SPINACH SOUP	182		X	X	X			15 minutes	7 g	10 g
LAMB AVGOLEMONO	184	X		X	X			14 minutes	4 g	5 g
LEBANESE HASHWEH	185	X	X		X			8 minutes	8 g	11 g
NAKED WONTON SOUP	187	X		X				10 minutes	2 g	2 g
PORK BELLY CABBAGE SOUP	188	X	X	X				15 minutes	7 g	9 g
PORK CHILE LETTUCE CUPS	191	X	X	X				15 minutes	2 g	3 g
PORK CHOPS AND CABBAGE WITH MUSTARD CREAM SAUCE	192		X	X	X			15 minutes	6 g	8 g
REUBEN CASSEROLE	194			X	X			15 minutes	2 g	5 g
SAUSAGE AND BROCCOLI	195		X	X	X			10 minutes	6 g	9 g
SICHUAN PORK WITH BOK CHOY	197	X	X					15 minutes	7 g	9 g
SKILLET LASAGNA	198			X	X			17 minutes	7 g	7 g
STUFFED POBLANOS	202		X	X	X			6 minutes	10 g	11 g
TEXAS CHILI	203	X	X	X	X			10 minutes	6 g	7 g
UNSTUFFED DOLMAS	204	X	X		X			8 minutes	7 g	14 g
INDIVIDUAL MEATLOAVES	205			X	X			24 minutes	6 g	7 g
"APPLE PIE" COMPOTE	209		X	X	X	X		10 minutes	3 g	6 g
5-INGREDIENT ALMOND COOKIES	210			X	X	X		15 minutes	3 g	19 g
CARDAMOM CUPCAKES	213			X	X	X		25 minutes	3 g	14 g

RECIPE	PAGE	DAIRY FREE	EGG FREE	NUT FREE	SOY FREE	VEGETARIAN	VEGAN	COOK TIME	NET CARBS	TOTAL CARBS
CINNAMON PIE CRUST	214	X	X		X	X	X	8 minutes	1 g	6 g
ICED CARAMEL MACCHIATO	215		X		X	X		4 minutes	1 g	1 g
COCONUT CHOCOLATE BARK	216		X	X	X	X		5 minutes	0 g	32 g
GRANOLA	219	X	X		X	X	X	5 minutes	2 g	10 g
LEMON POUND CAKE	220				X	X		20 minutes	6 g	34 g
PEANUT PECAN BARS	223	X	X		X	X		2 minutes	6 g	11 g
PEPINO CON LIMON	224	X	X	X	X	X	X		5 g	29 g
STRAWBERRIES AND CREAM	227		X	X	X	X			8 g	25 g
STRAWBERRY JAM	230	X	X	X	X	X	X	5 minutes	0 g	1 g
PB&J SHAKE	231	X	X		X	X	X		4 g	12 g
ALL-PURPOSE MUSTARD DRESSING	233	X	X	X		X	X			
ASIAN PEANUT SAUCE	233	X	X			X	X			
AVOCADO TOMATILLO DRESSING	236		X	X	X	X		5 minutes		
CILANTRO-JALAPEÑO DRESSING	237		X	X	X	X				
TANGY TAMARIND VINAIGRETTE	237	X	X	X				2 minutes		
ETHIOPIAN NITER KIBBEH	238		X	X	X	X		30 minutes		
HOMEMADE GHEE	239		X	X	X	X		25 minutes		
ZHOUG	241	X	X	X	X	X	X			
CAJUN SPICE	242	X	X	X	X	X	X			
HARISSA	243	X	X	X	X	X	X	1 minute		
RAS AL HANOUT	243	X	X	X	X	X	X			
INDIAN GARAM MASALA	244	X	X	X	X	X	X			
TZATZIKI WITH TAHINI	244		X	X	X	X				

INDEX

NOTE: Page references in *italics* refer to photos of recipes.

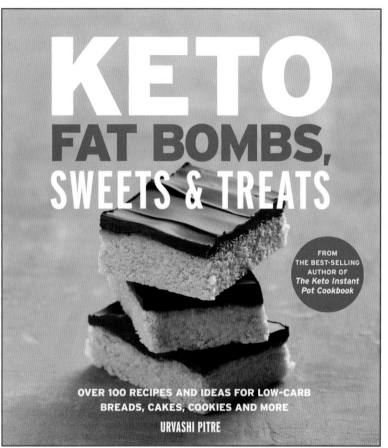
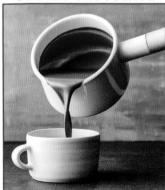
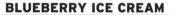
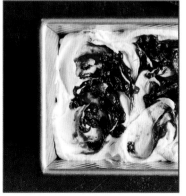
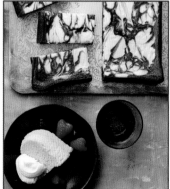

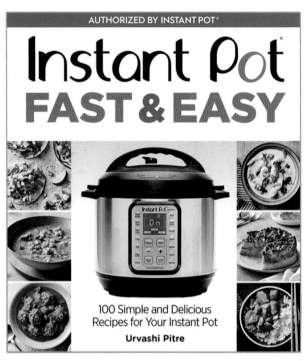
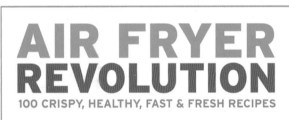

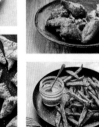
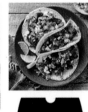
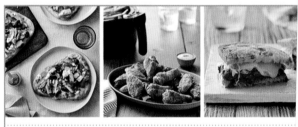
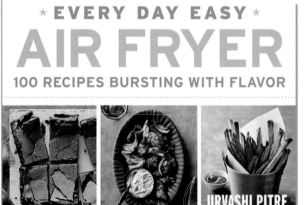